Communication Ski...

Final MB

Fines are chargeable on this book if you keep it beyond the agreed
date.
20p per day / £1 per week

This book is dedicated to our parents, without whom we would never have become doctors.

'This fellow's wise enough to play the fool;
And, to do that well, craves a kind of wit:
He must observe their mood on whom he jests,
The quality of persons, and the time;
And, like the haggard, check at every feather
That comes before his eye.'

Twelfth Night Act III Scene I by William Shakespeare

Commissioning Editor: Laurence Hunter
Development Editor: Janice Urquhart
Project Manager: Frances Affleck
Designer: Erik Bigland
Illustration Manager: Bruce Hogarth
Illustrator: David Banks

Communication Skills for

Final MB

A GUIDE TO SUCCESS IN THE OSCE

H.R. Dalton MB BS BSc DPhil(Oxon) FRCP DipMedEd
Consultant Physician, Royal Cornwall Hospital, Truro, UK

S.I.R. Noble MB BS MRCP PGCE DipPalMed
Senior Lecturer in Palliative Medicine, Cardiff University Medical
School, Cardiff, UK

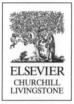

ELSEVIER
CHURCHILL
LIVINGSTONE

EDINBURGH LONDON NEW YORK OXFORD PHILADELPHIA ST LOUIS
SYDNEY TORONTO 2006

ELSEVIER
CHURCHILL
LIVINGSTONE

First published 2006

ISBN 0 443 10050 0

British Library Cataloguing in Publication Data
A catalogue record for this book is available from the British Library

Library of Congress Cataloging in Publication Data
A catalog record for this book is available from the Library of Congress

Notice
Medical knowledge is constantly changing. Standard safety precautions must be followed, but as new research and clinical experience broaden our knowledge, changes in treatment and drug therapy may become necessary or appropriate. Readers are advised to check the most current product information provided by the manufacturer of each drug to be administered to verify the recommended dose, the method and duration of administration, and contraindications. It is the responsibility of the practitioner, relying on experience and knowledge of the patient, to determine dosages and the best treatment for each individual patient. Neither the Publisher nor the authors assume any liability for any injury and/or damage to persons or property arising from this publication.

The Publisher

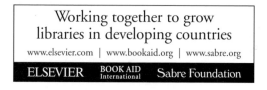
Printed in China

Preface

There is increasing awareness of the need to train tomorrow's doctors in communication skills. This is reflected in changes to the undergraduate curriculum and consequently the final examinations.

The communication skills stations in the OSCE are the most frequently failed by students and most dreaded by candidates coming up to finals. From our experience, even good students can fail these sections, not because they are bad communicators, rather they panic and say something stupid.

This book is not a book on how to communicate. It is a book focussed on getting you through the exam. Most people who fail these stations do so by making basic mistakes brought on by nerves or (in the case of history taking stations) poor knowledge of the basic facts.

The strengths of this book are as follows:

- It focusses on real examination questions
- The most common reasons for failing each scenario are looked at in detail. If you avoid these mistakes you are halfway there to passing!
- Model consultations are included with a commentary to explain the communication techniques being used.
- Numerous fact sheets are included which cover essential information required for passing the history-taking stations and help you remain focussed.

The style of the book is deliberately informal. The authors have over 25 years undergraduate teaching experience and are regularly involved with communication skills training and assessment. We know the secrets and pitfalls and have written this book with regular feedback from students, examiners and actor patients.

It is written as a companion to the best selling *Final MB*, which we recommend to you.

H. R. D.
S. I. R. N.

v

Acknowledgements

We are also grateful to the following people for their support and feedback in the preparation of this manuscript: Barbara Noble, Colin Kerrigan, Victoria Wheatley, Emma Mason, Claire Job, Colin Perdue, Jennifer Philips, Judith Johnson-Horner, Julie Rowlands, Meg Williams, Melanie Jefferson, Bethan Jones, Laurence Hunter and Janice Urquhart.

Contents

PART 1

INTRODUCTION

1

The most important chapter in the book!

This book does not aim to teach you how to communicate. Its prime aim is to teach you how to pass the exam.

Very few candidates fail the exam because they are bad communicators in real life. They fail because they perform badly in the exam. In the same way that there are certain rules and actions that must be followed in order to pass a driving test, so must you be seen to do all the right things in your communication skills exam. Many students come out of the exam feeling the examiners didn't get a realistic idea of how they normally communicate.

Lets face it; you are being assessed on an everyday skill in an extremely artificial environment. You are given a fixed time to take a specific history from actor-patients (of varying authenticities) whilst two examiners look on. It's so artificial; no wonder people go to pieces. No matter how competent you are at talking to patients, you could still flunk the exam without a strategy.

The primary aim of this book is to teach you how to pass an unfair exam. Whilst the bulk of advice is given to help you score the necessary points to pass, hopefully the things you learn from it will rub off and help you be a better communicator.

HOW TO PASS

Avoid sure fail mistakes

An important point to be aware of is that candidates who fail, tend to fail themselves by doing something truly bad. This tends to happen in the heat of the moment, when panic sets in. We panic. We do something stupid. We fail.

An important aspect of the exam must therefore be to avoid doing sure fail things. If you avoid them you are halfway there.

Each section of the book will outline common pitfalls to avoid. We have illustrated them with examples so you may better understand why and how these pitfalls should be avoided. If you can see the consequence of saying something silly, you are more likely to remember not to do it.

There are some generic pitfalls that must be avoided at all costs.

Danger! Common pitfalls

- ✘ Not introducing yourself.
- ✘ Not checking a patient's prior knowledge.
- ✘ Use of jargon.
- ✘ Being rude or dismissive to a patient.
- ✘ Ignoring obvious cues that there is another agenda to be discussed.

These are all pretty straightforward really, but easily forgotten when nerves set in.

Have a strategy when you can't think of what to say

It is almost inevitable that at some point your mind will go blank and you won't know what to say next. Panic then sets in. The more you try to think of something the worse it gets. There are several things you can do when this happens. All of them will buy you extra thinking time and, since they are valid communication techniques, they may even get you extra marks!

1. Listening skills

Listening skills are an essential part of the consultation. In the exam we tend to feel uncomfortable if there is a silence, but allowing time for the patient to ask a question or respond to information is important. Also don't forget that the actor-patient will want to fill the silence and will do so if given the opportunity.

Sometimes listening can be augmented by encouraging the patient to carry on talking with encouragements such as: 'I see', 'Yes', 'Go on', etc. Do not be afraid of silence. The patient will talk if given the opportunity.

Doctor:	How have you been feeling?
Patient:	Terrible doctor. I have been having awful tummy pains.
	(Panic sets in. You can't remember how to take a pain history.)
Doctor:	I see.
Patient:	Well it's low down and comes and goes.
	(Silence)
	It's a really crampy pain doctor.
Doctor:	Go on.
Patient:	I don't know what to do with myself when it comes on. Nothing seems to help.
	(After a few seconds of thinking time this has prompted you to remember to ask about exacerbating and relieving features.)
Doctor:	Does anything make the pain worse?

2. Recapping

Another trick if your mind has gone blank or you don't know what to say next is to recap. By going back over the patient's story, you are demonstrating that you have been listening. It offers the patient a chance to clarify anything you have missed. Often the patient will then pick up on something and direct your consultation for you.

Doctor:	Let me just recap what you've been telling me, Mr. Hull. From what I understand you have noticed that you have been losing weight and you've found it difficult to swallow.
Mr. Hull:	That's right doctor. What do you think it is?

This will hopefully prompt you to discuss possible diagnoses or ask a few more questions. Another technique with recapping is to ask if there is anything else the patient has noticed. Don't forget the actor-patient may give you extra information if you do this.

> **Doctor:** Let me just recap what you've been telling me, Mr. Hull. From what I understand you have noticed that you have been losing weight and you've found it difficult to swallow.
>
> **Mr. Hull:** That's right doctor.
>
> **Doctor:** Have you noticed anything else that you think might be related?
>
> **Mr. Hull:** I'm not sure if its relevant but I have been getting a lot of indigestion recently.

3. Reflecting

Reflecting back what a patient has said to you is a useful tool to buy you some thinking time if your mind goes blank. It is seen by the patient as encouragement to carry on talking and demonstrates that you have been listening.

> **Mrs. Scott:** I've been feeling tired all the time doctor.
>
> **Doctor:** *(Pause)* Tired all the time?
>
> **Mrs. Scott:** Yes. I'm normally full of life but ever since I lost my husband I've had no energy.

4. Checking

Often when discussing complex or distressing issues with patients, it is important to stop and check how the patient is doing. It demonstrates empathy, gives you time to think, encourages dialogue and can help guide the consultation. It is an essential technique in breaking bad news but is very effective for when your mind goes blank.

> **Doctor:** Now, that's a lot of information to take on board in one go, Mr. Hull. How has it left you feeling?
>
> **Mr. Hull:** To be honest doctor I feel numb.
>
> **Doctor:** It must be an awful shock for you.
>
> **Mr. Hull:** It is doctor. What do we do now?

5. Medicines

If in doubt talk about medicines! Any history-taking scenario will require questions about medicines. Since all medicines have side-effects, it is sensible to take a medicine history to see if any can account for the patient's presentation.

Know some facts

There is no easy way around this. You need to have a basic grasp of the relevant facts before you can communicate them. No short-cut here, you have to learn it. Although we cannot make you learn the facts we have provided you with relevant fact sheets covering essential information on each topic. This information is not exhaustive but will help you on the way.

Spend time with patients

A common comment we hear from examiners at Finals time is:

> 'You can tell after two minutes whether the student has spent time with patients at all'

The way you approach a patient, the level of discomfort you demonstrate, the rapport you develop are all tell-tale clues that the examiner picks up on. The rapport you build with a patient can sometimes direct how the consultation goes. If you are surly and the actor-patient takes a dislike to you, you may find the answers less forth-coming, with less information being spontaneously volunteered.

Don't forget. The reason most people want to become doctors is to help patients. Talking to patients is a privilege. Complete strangers trust us with their most private secrets, trusting us to try and help them. If you don't like spending time with patients, think carefully about why you are studying medicine.

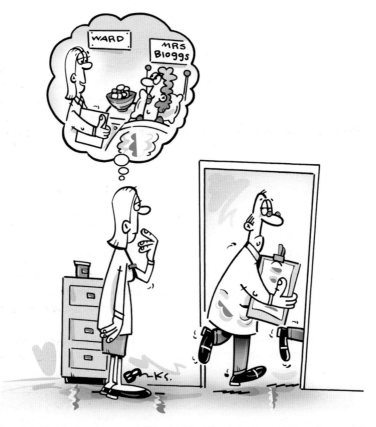

Fig. 1.1 'If only they saw me talking to Mrs Bloggs last week! Then they would have seen how good I can be.' The examination is an extremely artificial environment; people often go to pieces.

2

Different types of scenario

There are several generic communication skills that you will be required to demonstrate in every scenario you may come across. If you can't master these, you will struggle with the more complex cases. However, these skills are the sort you use every day and so unless you are completely socially inept you should be able to manage! Generic communication skills required in every consultation include:

- Checking the patient's prior knowledge or understanding.
- Listening.
- Avoiding the use of jargon.
- Eliciting and addressing the patient's agenda.
- Going at a pace that is comfortable for the patient.

If you work through the book in the order it is written, you will see a change in the balance between communication skills required and knowledge base. Early chapters require little factual knowledge but rely heavily on discussing difficult subjects.

The later chapters are impossible to tackle without a sound knowledge base. This is not to say that the later chapters require fewer communication skills. A consultation to elicit the cause of anaemia could quite easily turn into a consultation to discuss the possibility of cancer. By tackling the early scenarios first, you are likely to hone your generic communication skills, which are required for the later tasks.

DISCUSSING DIFFICULT SITUATIONS

These are covered at the beginning of the book since they rely on pure ability to communicate. Although little factual knowledge is required for these scenarios they are the most challenging since they are likely to illicit strong emotional responses from the actor-patient. We have found that people who fail these scenarios do so, not because they are poor at communicating but because they make glaring mistakes in the heat of the moment. These usually occur because they are nervous and panic. The skill to passing is therefore to avoid making glaring mistakes and to have basic strategies for when panic sets in.

Predominant skills required:

- Ability to discuss difficult situations.
- Listening skills.

Reasons candidates fail this scenario:

- Failure to check prior understanding.
- Use of jargon.
- Poor listening skills.
- Discomfort with patient/carers distress.

These are discussed in detail in the relevant chapters.

INFORMATION GIVING

These scenarios require you to transfer information and ensure that the patient understands what has been said. Often these scenarios involve discussions about sensitive or personal issues, and a professional approach is essential.

Predominant skills required:

- Factual knowledge.
- Ability to discuss difficult issues.

Reasons candidates fail this scenario:

- *Failure to check prior understanding*: if you assume patients know something, the chances are they don't and the consultation will go horribly wrong.
- *Use of jargon*: simple understandable words only.
- *Discomfort with discussing sensitive issues*: if you show you are embarrassed it will destroy any confidence the patient has with you.
- *Lack of factual knowledge*: you can't counsel someone on a subject you know nothing about.

DISCUSSING TREATMENT ISSUES

These scenarios require the candidate to impart information in a clear way to help patients decide on the best course of action in their care. The patient is likely to have concerns about the situation and you may be required to anticipate and manage these fears. Therefore, these scenarios are often the hardest since your agenda and the patient's may differ considerably.

Predominant skills required:

- Factual knowledge of subject.
- Ability to impart information.
- Listening skills.
- Ability to discuss difficult issues.

Reasons candidates fail this scenario:

- *Lack of factual knowledge*: if you don't know the subject you can't discuss it!
- *Use of jargon*: even if you know the subject, jargon prevents the patient from understanding it.
- *Poor listening skills*: failure to listen to the patient will prevent you from picking up on crucial concerns.

HISTORY TAKING

Pure history taking scenarios are usually the most straightforward. So long as you are familiar with the specialty in question, you should be able to ask the right questions. These scenarios may have an occasional additional challenge, such as a hidden agenda of the patient, but in general these scenarios are the easiest to pass.

Predominant skills required:

- Factual knowledge of differential diagnosis.
- Ability to take focussed history.
- Awareness of specific issues.

Reasons candidates fail this scenario:

- *Lack of factual knowledge*: if you don't know the causes of pyrexia of unknown origin, how can you take a history on it?

- *Inability to focus on the subject in question*: a full history is too time consuming for this exam. You must be able to focus on the most relevant areas of the history.

You will notice that the beginning of the book concentrates on several generic communication skills required for all consultations (and invaluable in sensitive discussion) and less on factual knowledge. As the book progresses, examples demonstrating generic communication skills diminish to be replaced more and more by facts. We make no apology for this. Hopefully, as you work through the book, the generic skills will become second nature to you and we will not need to go on about them. Just because we have not overemphasised the generic skills in the later chapters it does not mean they are any less important than the scenarios in the earlier chapters. We just don't want to bore you with too much repetition. There are some things we will 'drum into you' which we feel strongly about. If you find yourself sick of being told to 'check prior knowledge', we have done our job!

3

Different patient types

The actor-patients in the exam will be given a particular remit on how to behave. If your patient is angry in the exam, it is because that is part of the brief. Every student will get the same angry patient. If the patient doesn't stop talking and rambles off at tangents, this is all part of the exam, to test how you manage the consultation effectively. Sometimes a patient will be very quiet and unforthcoming with information. It is likely that the actor-patient has been told to behave this way for a reason, perhaps because of depression.

The actor-patient doesn't suddenly decide 'Aha! I fancy having a bit of a laugh! I know! I'll give the next student a hard time and pretend to be really angry!' The patient will be behaving according to the instructions from the examiners and for no other reason.

Obviously an actor-patient is told to behave in a certain way for a purpose. The important thing for you is to identify what features the examiners are looking for in your interaction with the patient. Once you have worked this out, you can conduct the consultation accordingly. We have outlined the four commonest types of 'difficult patient' (or relative) that you may encounter.

MR. ANGRY

The angry patient or relative is included in the exam because it is a common situation faced by healthcare professionals. If handled incorrectly, 'Mr. Angry' will transform into 'Mr. Even More Angry Than Before'. Students find angry consultations difficult because angry people are usually so wound up that they have lost all rational thought. They don't want satisfactory answers; they have gone beyond that point. They just want someone they can take their frustration out on. That happens to be you.

Avoid doing the following at all costs:

- Get defensive.
  'Look! Don't blame me! I'm not the doctor who normally looks after your mother!'

- Try and interrupt.

  'Okay, you've had your say. Now let me try and get a word in'

- Respond to anger with anger.

  'Listen pal. Don't get narkey with me. If I weren't wearing this white coat, I'd take you outside for a good shoeing!'

- Correct factual errors.

  'Actually I did see your mother today. At 10.30 this morning actually'

- Try to get on his good side by colluding with his poor opinion of a colleague.

  'I agree with you! Doctor Grint is completely useless. I don't blame you for being hacked off!'

It is sometimes useful to understand Mr. Angry's perspective. He will feel that no-one listens to him, that no-one is doing anything, no-one is giving him the answers he wants and the only way to get this sorted is by getting cross. He will have wound himself up to this point and 'unwinding' him will require time and patience. His anger is not personal. You just happen to be the focus of it.

Useful strategies include:

- Don't take it personally.
- Listen to him. Allow him to rant. There is no point in trying to reason with him until he has done this. He will eventually burn himself out.
- Identify what issues need addressing. If you can deal with them; do so. If you can't, devise a plan to sort them out and outline this to the patient/relative.
- If the consultation completely breaks down, suggest that both parties have a break and resume the conversation in ten minutes time. (This is very unlikely to occur in the exam.)
- Be honest. If you don't have the answer, say so, but also demonstrate that you will get the answer for him.

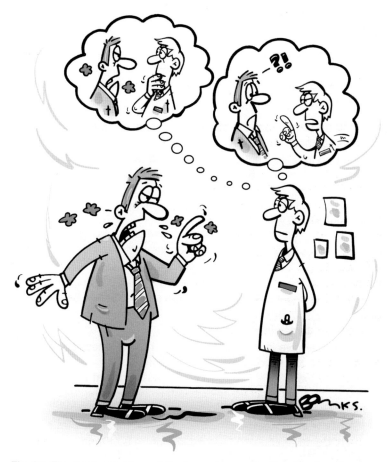

Fig. 3.1 The angry patient or relative is a common situation; handle with care.

MISS INCONSOLABLE

If you give people devastating news, they will respond with appropriate distress. They will cry, they will scream they will be unable to focus on anything. You will read later in the book the obvious, yet useful, saying:

'Bad news is bad news! You can't make it good news!'

In other words there is no easy way to give bad news and however you do it will be upsetting for the patient. The chapter on breaking bad news (Ch. 6) covers this in detail, but as a brief outline remember the following points when dealing with distressed people:

- Don't try and retract the bad news or change the severity of the news to cheer them up.
- Don't go into information overdrive and talk non-stop because you feel uncomfortable with the person's distress.
- Allow silence. Allow them to be upset.
- Encourage them to verbalise how they feel.
- Demonstrate empathy.
- Always, always, always end the consultation with some form of plan for the person to focus on.

MR. UNCOOPERATIVE

Mr. Uncooperative is the nightmare patient who doesn't say much. In the exam, you have to ask yourself 'why?'.

- He may be depressed.
- He may be scared that the information he gives will confirm bad news.
- He may incriminate himself by telling you things, e.g. epilepsy and driving.
- There may be a hidden agenda.

In this scenario, as before, you should start with open questions and encourage a dialogue. Try to find out his priorities and address these. If he has none, you should ask closed questions, focussing on your agenda. Do not forget to ensure that you aren't missing any obvious barriers to communication such as:

- The patient is deaf.
- The patient doesn't speak the same language as you.
- The patient has cognitive impairment.

MISS CHATTERBOX

Miss Chatterbox won't stop talking. The problem is that most of what she says is irrelevant to the presenting issue. Unfortunately, she feels that everything she is talking about is vital for you to know!

You have a few tasks here:

- Demonstrate listening skills.
- Allow dialogue so that the patient feels her story is being listened to. She may give you all the information you need, so don't interrupt too early.
- Demonstrate appropriate use of closed questions to get specific information.
- Keep her on the right track without offending her.

A good approach, having allowed her to talk for a while, is to say something like:

'It sounds like there are quite a few important things to discuss here. With your permission, I would like to ask you a few specific questions about each problem. After I've done that, if there is anything you think I have missed out, we can discuss them then.'

Another good pre-emptive line is:

'If at any point, I interrupt, I'm not doing it to be rude. It's just that there may be something very important I need to focus on. I hope that's okay with you.'

This should allow you to address her agenda but also give you permission to keep her 'on track' should she digress too much.

Finally, it is worth remembering that most scenarios will be straightforward. Only a few will involve patients with specific remits on how to behave.

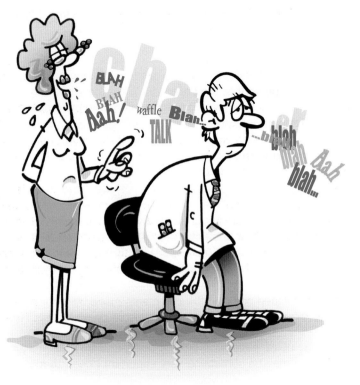

Fig. 3.2 Information overload; use your listening and questioning skills to filter out the useful points.

4

The actor-patient's perspective

Most medical schools use actor-patients for their communication skills examinations. In the past, they have varied in authenticity, with some truly awful over-acting. The quality of actor-patients that you are likely to encounter now will be very good. Medical schools tend to use the same individuals for the exam each time and students report them to be very authentic.

Usually these actors are professional actors who specialise in communication skills training and often will have been involved in your training during the year. Others may not be professional actors but are involved in the healthcare profession and familiar with the dynamics of a consultation.

As part of the preparation for our book we have interviewed several actor-patients for their views on what is necessary to pass the exam. Their views are important and valid since many will advise the examiners on how they feel a candidate performed. It is not unusual for examiners and actor-patients to mark candidates and compare for validity. Ninety-five per cent of the time their marks are the same!

We have collated some of the comments made by actor-patients interviewed and arranged them under relevant sub-headings. These are direct quotes from people who know!

FIRST IMPRESSIONS

'The first impression is so important. The way the student greets you can determine how the rest of the consultation will go.'

'Before the patient comes in, think about how you are going to introduce yourself and start off. Think to yourself; "How am I going to greet this person?"'

'Often students will just reel off the lines: "Now what seems to be the problem?" or "How can I help you?" The problem is it sounds "too taught", like you haven't thought about what you are going to say. As a patient, it feels like you can't be bothered. You haven't made the introduction your own.'

WHAT MAKES A GOOD STUDENT

'A good student is one who comes across as empathic. Not only do they appear to care but they also understand.'

'Good use of recapping and reflection are important. It really makes the patient feel you are listening to them.'

'Just by recapping with: "So what you're saying is . . ." makes you feel that you are being taken seriously.'

'Proper use of open and closed questions is important. Open questions are necessary to allow the patient to tell their story. Sometimes as an actor you have a brief that you are shy and will only give a decent history if a student asks the correct closed questions. In that situation, if I'm asked open questions I will give monosyllabic answers.'

USE OF SILENCE

'If you give a patient bad news or a lot of difficult information, it is inevitable that there will be silence. You will hear silence, but for the patient opposite you there is nothing but noise. It's just all internal. They need a bit of time to sort it out in their head and if you talk too soon during the silence, it will interrupt them.'

'Silence is okay. It doesn't come across that you don't know what you are doing. Give them loads of time, loads of space. Sit back and let them get it all right in their head.'

EYE CONTACT

'Eye contact is important to do but the student also needs to know when not to do it.'

'For a shy patient too much eye contact is intimidating. Do not stare them down. Many patients will be emotional and will not make eye contact.'

PRACTICE! PRACTICE! PRACTICE!

'You can soon tell if someone hasn't done much role-play. If you are uncomfortable with role-play, don't run away from it. Force yourself to practice. Practice with your friends. It's much better to make your mistakes in front of friends rather than the examiners.'

USE OF TOUCH

'The use of touch is very individual. Some students feel comfortable using touch to offer comfort. Touching on the shoulder or side of the arm is acceptable but be careful with touching the knee.'

'The use of touch comes naturally to some people, whilst to others it feels uncomfortable. You can spot these people a mile off. It looks so stilted. It looks like they're doing it because they think they should be. The consultation should flow naturally and not appear like you are doing it like a robot.'

ENDING THE CONSULTATION

'It is always good to end the consultation by summing up. Don't forget to check if the patient has anything they want to ask or add. It's important since it will allow the patient to direct to any agenda that you may have missed.'

5

Marking schedules

We are not going to spend too much time on marking schemes, since a knowledge of their intricacies is unlikely to help you much in passing the exam. We are mentioning them for completeness so you can use them as an outline when practicing scenarios.

There is no standardised marking schedule across all the medical schools. There are similarities, however. Some are very rigid as to how the examiner can score a performance, whilst others are more flexible, allowing examiners to give a mark based on an overall impression. Schedules are likely to vary according to the scenario. For example, a history taking station will have a larger proportion of marks allocated to obtaining information rather than generic communication skills, whilst a breaking bad news consultation will focus almost entirely on generic communication skills.

Although marking schedules vary, there appears to be ten core features similar to all of them. We have attempted to outline these below:

- Introduction/greeting.
- Checking patient understanding.
- Body language.
- Open questions then closed questions.
- Facilitate patient dialogue: head nodding, etc.
- Pace and flow of consultation
- Use of jargon.
- Addressing a patient's views/agenda.
- Demonstrating empathy.
- Summary/finishing with a plan.

These are graded differently. Most Schools give scores for each section out of 3 or 5 depending on performance.

Out of 5:
1 = poor, 2 = fair, 3 = average, 4 = good, 5 = excellent

Out of 3:
0 = Not done/ not done appropriately

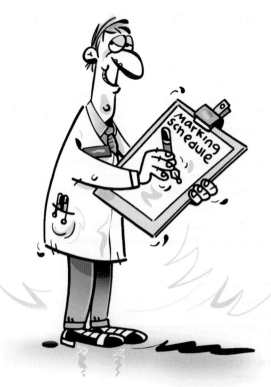

Fig. 5.1 Some marking schedules are very rigid; others are more flexible, allowing examiners to give a mark based on an overall impression.

1 = Done adequately
2 = Done appropriately and completely

Some marking schedules are more prescriptive and detail what key features need to be elicited. For example, when allocating marks for 'Addressing patient's views/agenda', examiners may give specific criteria needed to gain marks.

Mark	Criteria
0	Demonstrates no attempt to identify patient agenda Shows no interest in patient concerns Does not address patient concerns in any way
1	Identifies very little of the patient's agenda Shows minimal interest in patient concerns Addresses very few patient concerns
2	Partially explores and identifies patient agenda Demonstrates some understanding and empathy but misses major issues Addresses some patient concerns but does not fully reassure patient
3	Explores and identifies patient agenda Demonstrates understanding and empathy with regards to major patient issues Addresses most but not all patient concerns
4	Fully explores and identifies patient agenda Clearly demonstrates understanding and empathy Fully addresses patient concerns

To be honest there isn't much difference between this schedule and the mark out of 5.

The history taking scenarios will have specific information that the examiners will expect you to elicit. We have attempted to cover these in the fact sheets at the end of each chapter and have included a list of essential questions.

PART 2

DISCUSSING DIFFICULT SITUATIONS

6

Breaking bad news: the basics

By now you are probably sick of lectures on how to break bad news. You've had your fill of 'actor-patients' crying at the appropriate moments in the simulated consultation and you've had so many recorded consultations that you are thinking of opening up a video store. So this section is not going to teach you what you already know. It is going to cover the essentials but concentrate on the areas where candidates most commonly make their mistakes in the exam.

Let's first recap on the 10 steps in breaking bad news:

1. Preparation

- Know all facts before meeting.
- Who does patient want present?
- Ensure no disturbances: leave bleep with someone.
- Enough chairs are available for everyone: in a private setting.

2. What does patient know?

- Assess what they understand is happening at the moment.
- Ask for their narrative of events.
- Gives you an idea of how much they know, vocabulary etc.

3. Is more information wanted?

- Test the waters.
- Be aware that it may be frightening to ask for more information.
- 'Would you like me to explain a bit more?'

4. Give a warning shot

- 'I'm afraid it looks rather serious.'
- Allow time for patient to respond.

5. Allow denial

- This is a powerful coping mechanism.
- It allows the patient to control the amount of information.

6. Explain (if requested)

- Narrow the information gap.
- Step by step.
- Detail will not be remembered. The way you do it will.

7. Listen to concerns

- Allows space for expression of feelings.
- 'What are your main concerns at the moment?'

8. Encourage ventilation of feelings

- This is vital as it conveys empathy.
- 'This must all have come as a bit of a shock for you.'

9. Summary and plan

- Summarise concerns, plan treatment, and foster hope.

10. Offer availability

- May need further information (details not remembered).
- May need support (adjustment takes weeks or months).

In the exam, breaking bad news is not just limited to telling people they are dying. It is whenever you give information to someone that may distress. Telling an old lady with syncopal attacks that she cannot drive may be devastating news, as she will lose her independence. A young girl with Crohn's may be horrified that her treatment will require steroids as this may lead her to put on weight. The principles are the same.

BREAKING BAD NEWS

Mr. Thomas Foley is a 62-year-old man admitted from clinic for investigation of painless jaundice. Ultrasound and subsequent ERCP have confirmed advanced carcinoma of the pancreas. CT scan of the abdomen shows it to be inoperable with extensive lymph node involvement. His outlook is poor with a life expectancy of months. You arrange to see him in his side room on the ward.

Danger! Common pitfalls

- ✗ Not checking prior knowledge.
- ✗ Use of jargon.

✗ Not allowing for silence.
✗ Discomfort with patient distress.
✗ Giving too much information too quickly.

Not checking prior knowledge

One of the commonest mistakes made in finals is not checking what the patient understands already about their condition. Do not assume anything. Just because one of your colleagues has documented that the patient has been fully informed about the possibility of cancer does not mean they have understood or retained the information.

Studies have demonstrated that patients can recall only 30% of what is said to them in a consultation so it is vital that you check beforehand what they know. Otherwise it has the potential to go very pear shaped indeed!

Doctor: Hello Mr. Foley.
Mr. Foley: Hello doctor.
Doctor: I've got the results of your biopsies.
Mr. Foley: Yes doctor.
Doctor: As you'll remember, Dr. Jones thought the scans looked highly suspicious and we needed to take some biopsies to confirm this. I'm afraid the results confirm that you do have cancer.
Mr. Foley: What! I had no idea!
(Mr. Foley becomes inconsolably distressed)

Likewise the patient may not wish to know all the news at once. It is important to check with the patient how much they want to know.

Doctor: Hello Mr. Foley
Mr. Foley: Hello doctor.
Doctor: How are you feeling today?
Mr. Foley: Just a bit nervous about my results really.
Doctor: What do you understand about what is going on at the moment?
Mr. Foley: Well, the other doctor told me the scans looked worrying and they needed to rule out cancer.

Use of jargon

Everyone is terrified of the word cancer and avoid using it at all costs. However it is important that by avoiding using the word doesn't lead to misunderstanding. The example below actually happened on a ward round.

Doctor:	Hello Mr. Foley
Mr. Foley:	Hello doctor.
Doctor:	Your histology shows that you have a mitotic lesion of the neoplastic variety.
Mr. Foley:	Thank goodness for that! For one awful moment I thought you were going to tell me I had cancer.

Likewise a too direct approach is not helpful. People will only hear the word 'cancer' in a sentence and be unable to take in any other information. A young girl on a ward round was told the news that she had early stage Hodgkin's disease. In practical terms this could be construed as good news since it is almost always curable. However, it is still a massive shock with many psychological implications and breaking this news should be done in a sensitive manner, not as once witnessed below.

Doctor:	Mrs. Jones?
Mrs. Jones:	Yes.
Doctor:	You have cancer, but it is a good cancer!
	(Mrs. Jones husband takes a swing at doctor)

In practice it is best to use words that the patient is familiar with and often they will tell you the diagnosis themselves. By following the technique of firing 'warning shots' you can break the news gently using words they understand or volunteer.

Doctor:	I'm afraid the results are not good.
	(Pause)
Mr. Foley:	Oh dear. What's wrong doctor?
Doctor:	I'm afraid the tests show an abnormality.
	(Pause)

Mr. Foley:	What sort of abnormality?
Doctor:	It shows that you have a mass in your pancreas.
	(Pause)
Mr. Foley:	A mass?
Doctor:	Yes, a growth of some sort.
	(Pause)
Mr. Foley:	Is it a tumour doctor?
Doctor:	Yes. It is a tumour.
	(Pause)
Mr. Foley:	How serious is it doctor?
Doctor:	I'm sorry but it does look serious.
	(Pause)
Mr. Foley:	Oh dear. Is it cancer doctor?
Doctor:	Yes Mr. Foley I'm afraid it is cancer.
	(Pause)

Not allowing for silence

The problem with this exam is that when we get nervous, we get verbal diarrhoea. If there is a pause we feel we have to fill the painful silence with more information or an inane comment. Do not do it!

Silence is a valuable tool in communicating. It helps by:

- Allowing the patient time to assimilate the news.
- Demonstrating to the patient you are listening.
- Giving the patient time to react.
- Giving the patient time to ask questions.

Imagine if the above consultation was done without allowing time for patient responses.

Doctor:	You have a mass in your pancreas, a growth of some sort. It's a tumour and it looks serious. Its cancer.
Mr. Foley:	Gulp.

The perfect consultation should have more listening than talking by the candidate. Next time you practice a consultation, have a friend time how much of it is spent by you talking and how much listening.

Discomfort with patient distress

'Bad news is bad news! You can't turn it into good news!'

Some doctors feel that they have broken news well because the patient didn't cry when they were told they had cancer. It is most likely that the patient didn't understand what was being said.

Bad news is bad news! By definition it is going to upset the receiver. If a patient cries, then they are expressing appropriate emotion for devastating news. It is normal to be upset by upsetting news and as professionals we need to be more comfortable with it. The problem is we feel guilty that we have made them cry and may feel compelled to say something to make it better.

Doctor:	I'm afraid you have cancer of the pancreas. *(Mr. Foley breaks down crying. Candidate shuffles uncomfortably)*
Doctor:	Don't cry. I'm sure it will be all right.
Mr. Foley:	Will it?
Doctor:	Of course it will. I'm sure the oncologist will be able to give you some chemotherapy to shrink the tumour so don't worry.

Mr. Foley will now go home thinking that although he has cancer, it is treatable. Treatable to a patient means curable. As time moves on and he gets no better he is going to get angry with the oncologists who aren't making him better. He will be even angrier when he is told that he is dying. He may even go into denial. He will be angry that he hasn't used this time getting his affairs in order, spending quality time with his loved ones instead of being in hospital receiving chemotherapy. His family's bereavement may be complicated as they felt lied to. All because someone couldn't handle a patient being appropriately distressed at distressing news.

When giving bad news allow time for the patient to react. If there has been a long silence don't wade in with more information. The patient is still trying to deal with the last bit of news. If you feel the need to say something offer some empathy or prompt for them to express their feelings.

Doctor:	This must all have come as a massive shock to you.
Mr. Foley:	I can't believe it.

Giving too much information to quickly

The main task in breaking bad news is taking a patient from a point where they know nothing to fully understanding everything, if they so wish to do so. The skill is in slowing down the transition of information so that the patient can handle it. Too much too soon will lead to psychological disarray and provoke denial.

The warning shot technique helps the candidate test the water and see how much the patient will allow them to tell.

Below is an example of someone breaking bad news to Mr. Foley properly. Every patient is an individual, and his or her response to news will differ. This consultation tries to demonstrate the most important communication techniques you will need to demonstrate in the exam.

Example answer

Consultation	Commentary
Doctor: Hello Mr. Foley **Mr. Foley:** Hello doctor.	Introduction, making sure you are talking to right person.
Doctor: How are you today?	Establishing rapport.
Mr. Foley: A bit nervous really. Worrying about my results.	
Doctor: You've been through a lot recently haven't you?	Displaying empathy.
Mr. Foley: Yes I have.	
Doctor: What do you understand about what has been happening to you recently?	Checking prior understanding.
Mr. Foley: Not much really. My G.P. saw me because I had become jaundiced. When I came to clinic they admitted me straight away and did lots of tests.	Allowing patient narrative so you can judge which words you can use with patient and finding out how much he knows
Doctor: Did anyone explain what they thought might be going on?	Clarifying what said before.
Mr. Foley: They did but to be honest I was so nervous that I've forgotten most of it. They said something about a blockage of my bile duct.	

Doctor: Would you like me to explain a bit more about what's going on?	Checking to see if more information wanted.
Mr. Foley: Yes please.	
Doctor: The blockage was caused by an abnormality in your pancreas.	Warning shot.
Mr. Foley: The pancreas. That's it. They said it was something to do with the pancreas.	
Doctor: It looks like the abnormality is quite a serious one.	Further warning shot. Pausing to allow response.
Mr. Foley: Oh . . . I see. What sort of abnormality?	
Doctor: I'm afraid the blockage is caused by a lump in your pancreas.	Further shot, slowly revealing the seriousness of things at pace patient can handle.
Mr. Foley: A lump?	
Doctor: Yes, a growth of some sort.	Getting nearer to euphemisms of cancer.
Mr. Foley: Oh dear. That does sound serious.	
(Doctor pauses)	
Mr. Foley: What sort of growth is it? It isn't cancer is it? Please don't let it be cancer.	Patient wants to know. Use of word cancer suggests it's something he has been thinking about.
Doctor: I'm so sorry Mr. Foley but it is a cancer. *(Pause)*	Must be honest now.
(Doctor allows Mr. Foley to take in news)	Allow time.
Doctor: This must have come a terrible shock to you.	Encourage ventilation of feelings and express empathy.
Mr. Foley: It has. I can't believe it's happening.	
(Pause)	
Mr. Foley: So am I going to need an operation?	Suddenly we need to go back to breaking bad news again and may have to tell him it's incurable if the talk goes that way.
Doctor: I'm afraid an operation wouldn't be able to help.	Warning shot.
Mr. Foley: Oh.	

Doctor: An operation wouldn't be able to take the cancer away.	Clarifying.
Mr. Foley: *(silence)*	Allow silence.
Doctor: I will ask one of my colleagues, Dr. Feenan, to see you. He is a cancer specialist and may be able to offer some chemotherapy.	Offer plan, some hope.
Mr. Foley: And that will get me better?	Bargaining.
Doctor: The chemotherapy will try and slow the cancer down. *(Pause).* I'm afraid it won't get rid of the cancer completely.	Warning shot again. Empathic way to deliver bad news.
Mr. Foley: It won't?	
Doctor: No. I'm sorry it won't.	Empathy.
Mr. Foley: What do you mean?	
Doctor: The treatment won't be able to cure you of the cancer.	Clarify again.
Mr. Foley: Am I going to die doctor?	He's asked a direct question.
Doctor: Yes. I'm afraid that you are.	Therefore a straight answer sympathetically given.
Mr. Foley: *(silence)*	Don't be afraid of silence!
Doctor: *(silence)*	
Mr. Foley: So what happens now? How long have I got?	
Doctor: How do you mean Mr. Foley?	Clarify what he means.
Mr. Foley: How long have I got to live doctor?	
Doctor: The honest answer is that I don't know.	The truth!
Mr. Foley: You must have some idea doctor. There are things I need to do.	He needs to make plans and we know at best guess that people with inoperable pancreatic cancer usually live for 3–6 months.
Doctor: I don't think we are talking about years.	
Mr. Foley: Not years?	
Doctor: I think we are talking less than that.	Warning shots again.
Mr. Foley: How long?	

Doctor: I think we are talking months.

Mr. Foley: Oh. (pause) Well thank you for being straight.

Doctor: I think it's important for us to concentrate on living with as best quality of life we can for you.

Now it is vital to agree on a plan and foster some hope.

Mr. Foley: Yes.

Doctor: I would like you to see Dr. Feenan and discus whether he thinks some chemotherapy might help slow the cancer down a bit

Another opinion but setting realistic goals. Reiterate what was said before.

Mr. Foley: Ok doctor.

Doctor: I would also like you to stay in contact with my specialist nurse Jill who works as part of the team. She can go through things we've discussed and answer any questions you may have.

Use of clinical nurse specialist vital (Also shows the examiner you are embracing a multidisciplinary approach to patient care)

Mr. Foley: Yes.

Offering further support.

Doctor: Do you have any questions at the moment?

Offer chance to ask questions.

Mr. Foley: To be honest my mind is blank. I'm sure I'll have plenty of questions when I go.

Doctor: If you do, write them down and ask Jill them. I'd be happy to see you to discuss anything else you wanted to ask.

Opportunity to discuss again

Offer availability.

Mr. Foley: Thank you.

Doctor: When is your family coming to see you?

Don't forget other people will be affected by this devastating news.

Mr. Foley: Later today.

Doctor: Would you like me talk with them?

Offer availability.

Mr. Foley: Yes. If you don't mind.

Doctor: Not at all. I'll ask the ward to call me when they arrive. Perhaps then if you have thought of any questions we could go through them then.

Finish consultation with a plan.

7

Discussing resuscitation status

Mr. Danny Edwards is a 72-year-old with no previous medical history. He was admitted three days ago with an extensive anterior myocardial infarction. During thrombolysis he had a VF cardiac arrest which required 200 joules shock. Yesterday he extended his infarction and received further thrombolysis.

Since then he has progressively deteriorated. He is hypotensive, anuric and has pulmonary oedema despite maximal inotropic support. The cardiologists feel there is no further active treatment available.

You have arranged to speak with his wife Julie to make her aware of how unwell he is. You will need to discuss his resuscitation status.

Essential skills required

- Sensitive and sympathetic approach.
- Knowledge of legal issues regarding Do Not Attempt Resuscitation (DNAR) orders.

Think list

Your objectives
- Inform wife of how ill her husband is (breaking bad news).
- Discuss resuscitation status.
- Agree with family that he should not be resuscitated.

Mrs. Edwards' issues
- Shock of how ill he is.
- Disbelief that nothing can be done.
- Desire to insist on resuscitation even if futile.
- Lack of understanding of what Cardio-pulmonary Resuscitation (CPR) entails.
- Feelings of guilt that if she agrees to DNAR it will be her fault that she 'allowed him to die'.

Danger! Common pitfalls

- ✗ Not checking prior knowledge.
- ✗ Rushing the consultation.

✘ Using medical jargon.

✘ Putting the onus on her to make the resuscitation decision.

This can be one of the hardest consultations to do. At least when we break bad news to the family of a patient who has been unwell for a long time, it comes as less of a shock. Mr. Edwards' wife is going to find it harder to take such grave news for many reasons:

- There was no warning for this. He was mowing the lawn 4 days ago.
- We can put a man on the Moon, so doctors should be able to get her husband better.
- He has already been resuscitated once so she will find it hard to accept that this cannot be done again.

Not checking prior knowledge

It is vital to ascertain what Mrs. Edwards understands about her husband's condition since he has deteriorated considerably since admission. You do not know what she has been told and how aware she is of his grave prognosis.

Doctor:	Hello Mrs. Edwards. I'm Dr. Jones.
Mrs. Edwards:	How's my husband, doctor?
Doctor:	When did you last visit him?
Mrs. Edwards:	I saw him yesterday. He didn't look at all well. The nurses said he was a bit worse.
Doctor:	You're right. He has been very unwell and things have been worse over the last few days.

If you assume she is fully up to date with his condition without checking, you risk delivering devastating news without preparing her for it.

Doctor:	Hello Mrs. Edwards. I'm Dr. Jones.
Mrs. Edwards:	How's my husband, doctor?
Doctor:	Well as you know, his heart attack was massive and his heart is now failing. Things have now taken a turn for the worse.
Mrs. Edwards:	Worse! I didn't even know he'd had a heart attack!

Rushing the consultation

As with breaking bad news, it is important to take things at the pace that Mrs. Edwards can cope with. She has a few issues to come to terms with in a short period of time and giving too much information too quickly will lead to psychological disarray. It is vital to allow time for each piece of information to sink in, elicit a response or generate questions. Rushing the consultation usually occurs when the candidate fails to allow for silence or opportunity for the patient to react.

Doctor:	I'm afraid your husband has taken a turn for the worse.
	(Pause)
Mrs. Edwards:	Oh dear.
Doctor:	His heart has become weaker.
	(Pause)
Mrs. Edwards:	Weaker?
Doctor:	Yes. His heart is failing.
	(Pause)
Mrs. Edwards:	Is he going to get better doctor?
	(Pause)
Doctor:	At the moment he is very poorly and I don't think he will get better from this.

If this information is given without pauses, it will be too much for the patient or relative to take the information in.

Doctor:	I'm afraid your husband has taken a turn for the worse. His heart has become weaker. His heart is failing. At the moment he is very poorly and I don't think he will get better from this *(Mrs. Edwards dissolves into a heap on the floor)*

Using medical jargon

Discussing a patient's resuscitation status is difficult and distressing for all involved. It is normal for families to show appropriate distress.

They may cry, scream, get aggressive or even just sit there. Often when faced with a distressed family we tend to get defensive and try to give too much information. We feel we need to cover ourselves legally and impart all the necessary information in order to convince loved ones of the grave outlook.

Unfortunately, when we get defensive, we tend to hide behind medical terminology. Candidates have been observed to give relatives full-on tutorials about the physiology of a failing heart. A distressed wife with no medical background does not need to be told about her husband's wedge pressure and systemic vascular resistance in order to understand that he is going to die!

Putting the onus on her to make the resuscitation decision

It is important to involve the next of kin in resuscitation decisions since it:

- includes them in their loved one's care
- allows them some control in what must seem a completely out of control situation
- prepares them for the likelihood that the loved-one is dying
- helps lessen a complicated bereavement.

It does not, however, mean that we should leave the decision solely up to the family in the vague hope that they will decide that DNAR is the best option.

The general public have a very distorted view of what cardiopulmonary resuscitation involves and the realistic outcome of a resuscitation attempt. Their understanding is greatly influenced by television where a majority of arrested patients will pull through, so long as George Clooney is on standby. Even a drowned patient washed up on a beach will come round, after two rescue breaths from Pamela Anderson, and be well enough to make the surprise beach barbecue that evening: no secondary pneumonia, no hypoxic brain damage.

The reality is sadly different. In Mr. Edwards' case, his heart is failing and nothing will improve this. The decision to not resuscitate is a medical one. Doctors are not obliged to instigate futile treatments and in this case, CPR would not be successful. Imagine if this was a patient who wasn't fit for an anaesthetic, insisting on an operation. There would be no issue with the doctor refusing to perform a futile operation that the patient had no hope of surviving. CPR is another medical intervention which, if futile, should not be instigated.

Try and see things from Mrs. Edwards' point of view for a moment. She can see that her husband is dying, and she will feel completely helpless to do anything about it. All she can do is visit each day and hope for the best. It is a very passive experience. He is given medicines via lines, hooked up to monitors and machines which the doctors and nurses fiddle with. She, his wife, can do nothing but sit there.

Doctor:	Yes. His heart is failing.
	(Pause)
Mrs. Edwards:	Is he going to get better doctor?
	(Pause)
Doctor:	At the moment he is very poorly and I don't think he will get better from this.
Mrs. Edwards:	Oh.
Doctor:	At the moment, we don't have a resuscitation decision on him. What would you want us to do if his heart stops?
Mrs. Edwards:	Resuscitate him at all costs!

Of course she is going to say resuscitate him! This is the one time she can be involved in his care and show that she loves him. Here she is, once helpless, now fighting his corner. Insisting the doctors go all out for her loved one is a useful way of her avoiding the issue that Mr. Edwards is dying. This has diverted attention from preparing her for his inevitable death onto futile treatments which he will not benefit from.

Asking relatives what should be done puts pressure on them to make an informed decision they are unqualified to make. Rarely will relatives decide against resuscitation since they will then feel responsible for the loved one's death since they 'allowed the doctors to let him die'.

Don't forget that the manner in which we prepare families for the death of a loved one will impact greatly upon their subsequent bereavement. Relatives who feels they allowed their loved one to die, will face their bereavement with added feelings of guilt, anger and helplessness.

Example answer

Consultation	Commentary
Doctor: Mrs. Edwards?	
Mrs. Edwards: Yes doctor.	
Doctor: I'm Dr. Stevens. I'm one of the doctors looking after your husband.	Checks correct relative and introduces self.
Mrs. Edwards: How is Danny?	
Doctor: When did you last visit him?	Check prior knowledge.
Mrs. Edwards: I saw him yesterday but haven't spoken to a doctor for a couple of days.	
Doctor: What have the doctors told you about Danny's condition?	Further clarification of what she knows.
Mrs. Edwards: Well I know he had a heart attack and that they gave him some clot-busting medicine.	
Doctor: Yes, go on.	Encourage dialogue.
Mrs. Edwards: I think he then became unwell and they had to shock him.	
Doctor: That's right.	So you have established how much she knows. Need to fire a 'warning shot' and so this question allows her to identify how ill he is.
Mrs. Edwards: That's about all I know.	
Doctor: How does he seem to you today?	
Mrs. Edwards: He looks really awful. What's happening doctor?	
Doctor: Well, as you said, Danny had a heart attack and we know it was a very big heart attack.	Recap what is known.
(Pause)	Many pauses to go at pace she can cope with. Allows time for clarification and questions.
During his treatment with clot-busting medicine, he became very unwell indeed *(pause)* and we had to restart his heart with an electric shock.	
(Pause)	
Sometimes people who have heart attacks can go onto have further heart attacks.	Further warning shot.

(Pause)	
Yesterday he became more unwell again.	Further warning shot.
Mrs. Edwards: What happened?	
Doctor: He had another heart attack, a big one, which has made his heart very weak indeed.	Further warning shot.
Mrs. Edwards: So what are you going to do for him?	
Doctor: We have got him on all the heart drugs there are to help with heart attacks.	Indicate maximal active treatment.
(Pause)	
He has been reviewed by the cardiologists, the heart specialists, and they agree that he is on all the right medicines.	To reassure that all is being done for him.
(Pause)	
Mrs. Edwards: I see.	
Doctor: Despite being on all the right medicines, his heart is still very weak.	Continue at pace she can manage.
(Pause)	
The second heart attack has made his heart so weak that it is having difficulty pumping.	
(Pause)	
That is why he looks so poorly today.	Reiterate how ill he is.
(Pause)	
Mrs. Edwards: But he will get better won't he?	
Doctor: Danny has had two big heart attacks and despite all the medicines he isn't improving. If anything he is getting more poorly.	Breaking bad news. Further warning shot.
(Pause)	
Mrs. Edwards: Oh.	
Doctor: I'm afraid that Danny is unlikely to get better from this.	
(Pause)	
Mrs. Edwards: He's going to die?	

Doctor: I'm very sorry Mrs. Edwards. Yes, I think Danny is going to die.	Honest answer with empathetic wording.
Mrs. Edwards: There must be something you can do.	
Doctor: He is on all the medicines possible to help his heart. Despite this, his heart is not getting better.	It is normal to go over things you have already covered.
Mrs. Edwards: I can't believe it. He was mowing the lawn 4 days ago.	Disbelief.
Doctor: It must be a terrible shock.	Empathy allowing further venting of feelings.
Mrs. Edwards: It is. I can't believe it. Are you sure there is nothing else that can be done?	
Doctor: Yes, we are sure. *(Pause)* The most important thing for Danny is to make sure he is comfortable.	Important to reaffirm the situation but talk about active process of symptom control.
Mrs. Edwards: Yes doctor. I don't want him to be in any pain.	
Doctor: We will make sure he won't be in pain.	
(Pause)	
I know that this must be awful for you, Mrs. Edwards. *(Pause)* It is important that we do what is best for Danny and not put him through any unnecessary procedures that won't help him.	Empathy. Go at a slow pace. When proceeding to talk about resuscitation status, the consultation needs to flow into it.
Mrs. Edwards: Yes.	
Doctor: If Danny's heart were to stop, I don't think we would be able to restart it again. *(Pause)* All the machines in the hospital wouldn't be able to restart his heart and even if they could, he would remain just as poorly. *(Pause)* His heart would stop again shortly after.	Identify futility of resuscitation and the medical decision not to attempt CPR.
Mrs. Edwards: But you restarted his heart when he came in.	Need to take time to explain why this time resuscitation will not work.
Doctor: That's right. His heart stopped because of an abnormal electrical rhythm in his heart.	
(Pause)	
His heart was stronger then before he had the second heart attack.	

(Pause)	
His heart is much weaker now and an electric shock wouldn't work in this case. It is not to do with electricity this time. It is because the muscle in his heart is worn out.	Use language she can understand. Do not be dismissive of her views.
(Pause)	
Mrs. Edwards: Oh.	
Doctor: It must be an awful lot to take in.	Empathy and opportunity to express feelings.
Mrs. Edwards: I don't know what to do now. Um. Should I call his brother? He has two children from his first marriage. Should I call them?	
Doctor: If there are people you feel it is important for Danny to see, then yes, I think you should call them.	Basically you are reiterating that he is dying and that this is likely to happen soon. Offer availability.
Would you like me to speak with them or would you like to do this yourself?	
Mrs. Edwards: I'll do it myself, thank you, doctor.	
Doctor: Okay. Is there anything else you want to ask or talk about at the moment?	Winding consultation up.
Mrs. Edwards: No. I don't think so. My mind has gone blank.	
Doctor: I am around if you need to talk about things or if you have any questions. I would just like to go and check that Danny is comfortable and then you can come in and see him if you like.	Offer availability.
Mrs. Edwards: Thank you doctor.	

This is basically a breaking bad news scenario, but this time you are breaking two pieces of news.

1. Mr. Edwards is going to die.
2. He will not be resuscitated.

Just because his wife has accepted the first piece of news, doesn't mean she will accept the second.

As in the first scenario (Breaking bad news, Ch. 6), it is important to anticipate and manage extreme expressions of emotion such as:

- anger
- disbelief
- tears
- screaming.

Don't forget that '**bad news is bad news and we can't turn it into good news**'.

It is normal for relatives to repeat the same questions, hoping that you may change the news you are giving. Painting a better outlook because you feel uncomfortable with their distress is the wrong thing to do.

PART 3

INFORMATION GIVING

8

Explaining a procedure/informed consent

The past few years have seen a major change in the way patients are consented for procedures. In the past, patients frequently signed consent forms with little or no understanding of the procedure or risks involved. In addition, they may have been consented by the most junior member of the team who often had about as much knowledge of the procedure as the poor patient!

In theory, the clinician providing the procedure should now obtain consent, but the General Medical Council Guidance states that the task of seeking consent may be delegated to another health professional, as long as that professional is suitably trained and qualified. This may still be a junior member of the firm.

Explaining an investigation is a common question in finals since it tests the candidate's knowledge of procedures and their general communication skills. Candidates will be expected to present information clearly, avoiding jargon, whilst demonstrating empathy that the patient is likely to be nervous. It is unlikely that they will be asked to actually consent the patient, but they should be familiar with the issues around consent.

To obtain *informed* consent, the following must occur:

1. Consent must be given voluntarily

Consent must be given freely by the patient, without pressure or undue influence on them to either accept or refuse the procedure. Such pressure can come from partners or family members, as well as healthcare professionals.

2. The person must be appropriately informed

To give valid consent, patients need to understand in broad terms the nature and purpose of the procedure. They should be informed of any 'material' or 'significant' risks in the proposed procedure, any alternatives to it and the risks of doing nothing. In theory, doctors should inform patients of any complications with a risk greater than 1 in 1000. In practice they should also mention rarer complications if they are considered serious.

3. The person must have the capacity to consent to the procedure

For a person to have capacity, he or she must be able to comprehend and retain information material to the decision. There should be an understanding of the consequences of having or not having the procedure, and the ability to use and weigh this information in the decision making process. Ideally, a patient should be consented well before the procedure, having had time to consider the information provided.

The Department of Health have published a set of guidelines in the document 'Reference Guide for Examination or Treatment' which can be downloaded (www.doh.gov.uk/consent/refguide.pdf); we strongly recommend you read this. We have given you a 'classic' finals question below with a model answer. At the end of this chapter (p. 58), you will find a set of fact sheets for procedures that have appeared in past exams.

DISCUSS WITH A PATIENT WHO IS DUE A BRONCHOSCOPY

Mr. David Gough is a 65-year-old, recently retired taxi driver. Four weeks ago he went to see his GP with a persistent cough and shortness of breath. After two courses of antibiotics his GP arranged a chest X-ray, which shows a suspicious mass in the right hilum. An urgent referral is made to the respiratory team and a bronchoscopy has been arranged. He arrives on the ward for a day-case bronchoscopy. You have been asked to explain the procedure.

Other ways this question has been asked would be with you as the GP, being asked to explain the results of Mr. Gough's chest X-ray and the need for a bronchoscopy.

Essential skills required

- Knowledge of what a bronchoscopy entails (see fact sheet, p. 58).

- Ability to put patient at ease.
- Use of non-medical jargon.
- Anticipate and manage pitfalls.

Think list

Your agenda	*Mr. Gough's agenda*
• Explain procedure to Mr. Gough.	• May not know why he is here.
• Ensure he understands procedure.	• Might be nervous of hospitals.
• Inform him of possible complications.	• Doesn't understand medical jargon.
• Explain that he will be consented for the procedure later.	

Danger! Common pitfalls

There are several common mistakes that students make that can be easily avoided:

✗ Not checking prior knowledge.
✗ Use of medical jargon.
✗ Addressing your agenda and ignoring Mr. Gough's.
✗ May have to discuss possibility of cancer (breaking bad news).

Not checking prior knowledge

Many disasters can be avoided by checking what the patient understands is going on. Even if the notes state that the patient has been informed of something, there will be nothing to suggest understanding or retention of the information.

Doctor:	Hello Mr. Gough. My name is Dr. Stevens.
Mr. Gough:	Hello doctor.
Doctor:	As you know, we need to do a special telescope test of your lungs.
Mr. Gough:	Why's that doctor?
Doctor:	Well, because of your chest X-ray. Anyway this test is called . . .
Mr. Gough:	Sorry doctor. What about my chest X-ray? Is there something wrong?

Doctor:	Well yes. Um. Didn't your GP tell you the result of it?
Mr. Gough:	No. I just got a letter telling me to come here today for a test. What is wrong with my chest X-ray doctor?

You can almost feel the doctor desperately trying to regain control of the consultation!

To avoid this, the candidate should check what the patient already knows about the procedure and why they are there.

Doctor:	Hello Mr. Gough. My name is Dr. Stevens.
Mr. Gough:	Hello doctor.
Doctor:	I've been asked to come and talk to you about a special test we would like to do. Has anyone spoken to you about this already?
Mr. Gough:	Not really doctor, no.
Doctor:	Well, we can talk about that in a moment. I gather, through your GP, you have been having problems with your chest.
Mr. Gough:	Yes doctor, etc. . . .

Use of medical jargon

Beware of using medical jargon!

Doctor:	It's a very simple procedure. I'll just *pop* a *cannula* in the *dorsum* of your hand and *administer* a small dose of *anxiolytic*. At the same time, we'll squirt some *'local'* down your nose and back of your *pharynx*. Once this is sufficiently *anaesthetised* well *pop* a small *fibre-optic scope per-nasally*, down the naso-pharynx past the cords and into the bronchial tree. We'll have a quick *scoot* around and *biopsy* anything abnormal. Complications are rare. A bit of *haemoptysis* is common.
Mr. Gough:	Pardon?

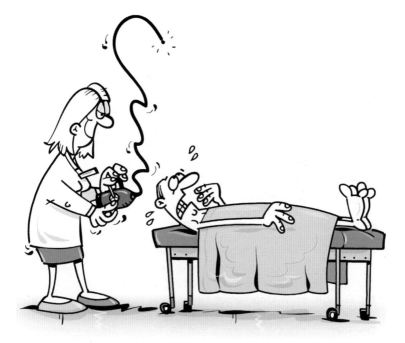

Fig. 8.1 Try to avoid medical jargon; the patient should understand the procedure to be performed.

We become so used to using medical words that we forget that most people have no understanding of such terminology. What's more, the majority of the general public have an average reading age of 12 and their vocabulary is likely to be limited. Practice consenting one of your non-medical friends for a procedure. You'll soon get an idea of how much you need to simplify things. See the 'model answer' below for words that can be used in the examination.

Addressing your agenda and ignoring Mr. Gough's

This is a common mistake in exams. You become so hell-bent on getting through the task of explaining the procedure that you ignore cues that might signal worries the patient is having.

A good tip is to acknowledge these concerns and agree to go back and discuss them a little later. This way you demonstrate to the examiner:

1. You have picked up on the patient's cues.
2. You have acknowledged their importance to the patient.
3. You are not going to ignore them.

One way of addressing a patient's concerns whilst addressing your agenda may be as follows:

Doctor:	First we will give you some medicine through a drip in the back of your hand. This is to make you feel a bit sleepy. Then . . .
Mr. Gough:	How long before I'll be back at work. I don't want to be off long!
Doctor:	I can understand that Mr. Gough. That's something that is obviously important to you and something we need to spend some time talking about. Would it be okay with you if we finish talking about the bronchoscopy and then we can concentrate properly on how this might affect work?
Mr. Gough:	Sure.

Discussing the possibility of cancer

We have seen candidates frozen solid in the exam when the patient has said one of the following:

'Is it something serious doctor?'
'What did my doctor mean by "shadow on the lung"?'
'So long as it isn't cancer I don't mind.'
'Since I've seen my GP I've coughed up some blood. What does that mean doctor?'

Some candidates have been livid since the question said 'consent for a bronchoscopy' and nothing about discussing cancer. However, lets not forget that we are consenting the patient for a test that may find cancer, and that the possibility of cancer being discussed is highly likely.

If this happens **do not:**

- Pretend you didn't hear it.
- Pass the buck for someone to talk about it.
- Ignore that the patient may be scared.
- Reassure unrealistically: 'I'm sure it'll be okay'.

Do:

- Acknowledge their concerns.
- Acknowledge that cancer is one of several possibilities.
- Stress the importance of having all the facts before making plans.
- Offer some realistic hope.

For further help on discussing cancer issues see Chapter 6.

Example answer

Consultation	Commentary
Doctor: Mr. Gough? **Mr. Gough:** Yes?	Checks correct patient and introduces self.
Doctor: Hello Mr. Gough. My name is Dr. Bloggs. I've been asked to come and talk to you about a special test we would like to do. Has anyone spoken to you about this already?	Check prior knowledge.
Mr. Gough: Not really. I was just sent a letter telling me to turn up here for an investigation.	
Doctor: I see. We can have a chat about that in a moment. Before we do that, would you mind telling me,	Reassure. Ask for patient narrative to see what they understand is going on and about to happen.

in your own words, what's been happening recently that has meant you coming here today.

Mr. Gough: Well, I've not been as well recently.

Doctor: In what way?

Shows you are listening.

Mr. Gough: Harder to breathe and an annoying cough. So I went and saw my GP who gave me antibiotics.

Doctor: I see. Did they help?

Encouraging dialogue.

Mr. Gough: Not really. He gave me stronger antibiotics but they didn't help either. So I went back to my GP and he sent me for a chest X-ray.

Doctor: And what did that show?

Listening.

Mr. Gough: I'm not sure. He said it was abnormal and that we needed to do some more tests. So here I am.

So he understands that he needs more tests but hasn't shown signs that he wants to know more.

Doctor: Did he mention anything about the test?

Mr. Gough: No nothing.

Doctor: Well your GP was absolutely right to refer you to us. As you say, your chest X-ray looks slightly abnormal and it is important that we take a closer look.

Reassure/ put at ease.

Words patient used.

Mr. Gough: Okay.

From now on lots of pauses by the candidate to allow the patient opportunity to ask questions.

Doctor: The test we would like to do is called a bronchoscopy. First we pop a small drip into the back of your hand and then give you some medicine, which will make you feel sleepy.

Non-jargon.

Mr. Gough: Yes.

Doctor: Then we will spray the back of your throat with some medicine to numb it. *(Pause)*.

Non-jargon.

We also squirt some jelly into your nose to numb things there as well.

Mr. Gough: Okay.

Doctor: We will then pass a small tube and a light into your nostril and then down into your windpipe. Don't worry it won't affect your breathing. *(Pause)*

With the tube and light, we will be able to have a close look around your lungs. It is usual for us to take some tissue samples so we can look at them under a microscope later.

Mr. Gough: Okay.

Doctor: You'll then come back to the recovery room for a few hours. You won't be able to drink at first because your throat will be numb and fluid might go down the wrong way. *(Pause)*

After a couple of hours the nurse will let you know when it's okay for you to go home. You might still be a bit sleepy, so it's important that someone else takes you home. Have you got someone to pick you up?

Mr. Gough: Yes. My wife is going to ring.

Doctor: Good. The bronchoscopy is a safe procedure but I need to tell you the commoner side-effects. It is quite common to cough up blood-stained phlegm for a couple of days if biopsy samples are taken. This is nothing to worry about and should clear up in a few days. *(Pause)*

If you continue to cough up blood or you think it is getting worse, then we need to know about it. The best thing to do is call your GP immediately. It is very rare indeed for there to be problems.

Doctor: Do you have any questions at all?

Mr. Gough: When will you know the results?

Time for response/questions.

Anticipate fears and reassure.

Lots of talking here.

Avoiding jargon.

Frequent pauses to check patient understands.

Informed consent.

You must tell patient of side-effects.

Important to give opportunity for questions.

Doctor: It normally takes about 5 days to get the results back. So we'll make an appointment for you to see us in clinic next week.	Follow-up plan important.
Mr. Gough: Okay.	
Doctor: The bronchoscopy will be done by Dr. Smith. He will be along soon to get your permission for the procedure. He will explain the procedure again and ask you to sign a consent form. Before you do this, I would ask you to read this information sheet. I'm afraid it's a bit long but it is important that you take time to read it. If you have any other questions after reading it, please feel free to ask before you sign.	

You will need to be flexible in your consultation. The patient may have specific fears that they want to discuss. Make sure you pick up on the cues!

Remember that the aim here is not just to impart information but also to make sure the patient has understood the information you have given.

On the next few pages we have fact sheets for other endoscopic procedures you may be asked to explain. Just follow the principles already covered and you should be fine.

Fact sheet: Bronchoscopy	
Facts you need to know	*Non-jargon ways to say it*
Indications • Investigation of suspected lung cancer • Biopsy of lesion on chest X-ray	This can only be done once you have an idea of the patient's prior knowledge. 'What do you understand about what's going to happen today?'
What procedure involves • Nil by mouth for 6 hours • Hyoscine and pethidine pre-med	'Nothing to eat for 6 hours.' 'We'll give you a pre-med injection which will relax you and may make

Fact sheet: Bronchoscopy—cont'd	
Facts you need to know	*Non-jargon ways to say it*
• Local anaesthetic sprayed into pharynx • Lignocaine gel nasally • Supplementary oxygen and saturation monitor	your mouth dry. We'll then spray the back of your throat to numb it and then squirt some jelly into your nose to numb things there as well.'
• Bronchoscope passed per-nasally past pharynx • Local anaesthetic sprayed onto vocal cords • Scope passed by cords and further local sprayed down each bronchus	'We'll then pass a small tube and a light into your nostril and then down into your wind-pipe. It might make you cough a little but won't interfere with your breathing.'
• Bronchoscope manipulated around bronchial tree. Biopsies, brushings and suckings taken as required • Procedure takes about 15–20 minutes	'The doctor will then have a close look around your lungs. It is usual for us to take some tissue samples so we can look at them under a microscope later.'
After care • Drowsy in recovery room • Nil by mouth for 3 hours • Must be picked up by someone • Not to drive, operate heavy machinery or drink alcohol for 24 hours	'You won't be able to drink at first because your throat will be numb and fluid might go down the wrong way.'
• Nosebleed and mild haemoptysis not uncommon • Results often given once patient awake but histology not available until clinic	'It is quite common to cough up blood-stained phlegm for a couple of days because of the tissue samples.'

Fact sheet: Upper gastrointestinal (GI) endoscopy	
Facts you need to know	*Non-jargon ways to say it*
Indications • Investigate suspected upper GI cancer • Investigate upper GI cause of anaemia, e.g. ulcer, cancer • Investigate upper GI symptoms, e.g. dyspepsia, dysphagia • Banding of oesophageal varices	Must first ascertain patient's understanding of why they are having test. Remember that they may have no idea that there is a chance of cancer, etc.

Fact sheet: Upper gastrointestinal (GI) endoscopy—cont'd	
Facts you need to know	*Non-jargon ways to say it*

What procedure involves
- Nil by mouth 6 hours
- Remove dentures
- Either throat spray or sedation

'We can perform the test using either throat spray, which numbs the back of the throat, or a sedative injection which will make you drowsy.'

- Lie on left side
- Mouth guard to protect teeth
- Endoscope passed orally
- Endoscope passed down oesophagus, stomach and duodenum

'A flexible tube will be passed through your mouth into your throat. It won't cause any pain or interfere with your breathing.'

- Air inflated to give better view

'Once inserted, air is passed into the stomach to give the doctor a better view.'

- Biopsies may be taken

'The doctor may want to take a sample of tissue, called a biopsy.'

- May feel bloated; suction often used during procedure
- Procedure takes 5–15 minutes

'If your mouth fills with saliva, the nurse will remove it with a sucker like at the dentist.'

After care
- If throat spray—nil by mouth for one hour
- If sedation—sleepy in recovery room
- Must be picked up by friend
- No driving, alcohol or operating heavy machinery for 24 hours (if sedated)

'If you have sedation, the sedative effects can last for up to 24 hours. It is important that a relative or friend comes to pick you up and can stay with you for 24 hours.'

Complications (less than 1:1000)
- Perforation
- Bleeding
- Reaction to sedative

'The doctors performing this test are trained endoscopists. Complications are rare (less than 1 in 1000) but there is a small risk of perforation or tearing of the intestine that could require surgery. *(Pause)* Rarely people can have a reaction to the sedative or have some bleeding after the procedure.'

Fact sheet: Upper gastrointestinal (GI) endoscopy—cont'd

Facts you need to know	*Non-jargon ways to say it*
Advise patient to call GP if they get • Signs of sepsis • Dysphagia • Increasing throat, chest or abdominal pain • Malaena	'You should contact your GP if you have any of these symptoms: fevers or chills, trouble swallowing, increasing throat or chest pain or notice that you are passing black tarry stools.'

Fact sheet: Colonoscopy

Facts you need to know	*Non-jargon ways to say it*
Indications Investigation of: • Altered bowel habit • Suspected bowel cancer • Inflammatory bowel disease • Rectal bleeding	Once again need to ascertain patient's understanding. Usually those coming for colonoscopy have had symptoms but it is always best to check.
What procedure involves • Bowel prep involving strong laxatives • Clear fluids day before colonoscopy • Remove undergarments • i.v. sedation • Lie left side with knees bent • Rectal examination • Pass colonoscope into rectum and then colon • Air to insufflate the bowel • Biopsies or polyp removal • Takes 15–60 minutes	'You should have been sent some bowel cleansing medicine to take before the test. This helps empty your bowels so the doctor can see things properly.' 'You will be asked to lie comfortably on your left side with your knees slightly bent. *(Pause)* The doctor will first examine the back passage with a finger and a glove. *(Pause)* The doctor will then pass a flexible tube into your back passage. *(Pause)* Air is passed through the tube to give the doctor a better view.' 'The doctor may wish to take a sample of the lining of your bowel.'
After care • Abdominal cramps/ bloating relieved by passing flatus • Sleepy in recovery room	'Cramped bloated feeling is usually relieved by passing wind.'

Fact sheet: Colonoscopy—cont'd	
Facts you need to know	*Non-jargon ways to say it*
• Someone to take patient home • Avoid driving, alcohol or operating heavy machinery for 24 hours	
Complications (less than 1:1000) • Perforation • Bleeding • Reaction to sedative	'The doctors performing this test are trained endoscopists. Complications are rare (less than 1 in 1000) but there is a small risk of perforation or tearing of the intestine that could require surgery. *(Pause)* Rarely people can have a reaction to the sedative or have some bleeding after the procedure.'
Advise patient to call GP if they get • Severe abdominal pain • Vomiting • Signs of sepsis • Continued bleeding	'You should contact your GP if you have any of these symptoms: severe abdominal pain, vomiting, fevers and chills or continued bleeding.'

Fact sheet: Endoscopic retrograde cholangio-pancreatography (ERCP)	
Facts you need to know	*Non-jargon ways to say it*
Indications • To image pancreas and bile ducts • Diagnosis of suspected pancreatic or biliary cancer • Stent placement in obstructive jaundice • Sphincterotomy	Check prior knowledge. It is highly unlikely that they have gone straight for an ERCP without other tests like an ultrasound.
What procedure involves Similar to endoscopy fact sheet but in addition: • Contrast media may be injected into bile duct and X-rays taken • Sphincterotomy	'A special dye is injected down the tube so that the pancreas and bile ducts can be seen on X-ray film.' 'Enlarge the opening of the bile duct with an electrically heated wire called a diathermy.'

Fact sheet: Endoscopic retrograde cholangio-pancreatography (ERCP)—cont'd	
Facts you need to know	*Non-jargon ways to say it*
• Stent placement • Procedure takes 15–60 minutes	'Short plastic bypass tube to allow bile to drain.'
After care • Recovery room then to ward • Usually overnight stay • Results given prior to discharge	
Complications For diagnostic ERCP: • 1–2% risk of pancreatitis • Contrast media reaction (rare) • Cholangitis (rare) For stenting or sphincterotomy: • 5% risk pancreatitis • 1% risk of bleeding from sphincterotomy site • 1% risk cholangitis • 0.3% risk perforation of intestine • 0.4% risk related mortality rate	'Inflammation of the pancreas.' 'Reaction to the injection dye.' 'Inflammation of the bile duct.'

Use of diagrams

Explaining a complex procedure like an endoscopy can often be improved by the use of simple diagrams. Do not be afraid to draw one for your patient as it will often aid their understanding of the spoken word.

9

Discussing a new medicine with a patient

Mrs. Jones was admitted with a right deep vein thrombosis (DVT), six weeks after a total hip replacement. She has been fully anticoagulated with warfarin and her INR is stable. She is going home today and you need to discuss her new medicine with her. She should remain on warfarin for three months.

Essential skills required

- Knowledge of warfarin pharmacology and practicalities (see fact sheets, p. 70 and 71).
- Ability to explain important information to patient.
- Use of non-medical jargon.
- Anticipate and manage barriers to patient compliance.

Think list

Your agenda
- Explain relevant details about new medicine.
- Optimise patient compliance.
- Inform her of possible side-effects and interactions.
- Explain follow-up plans.

Mrs. Jones' agenda
- May not understand why she needs the medicine.
- Doesn't like taking tablets.
- Feels better now, so what's the point of taking tablets.

Danger! Common pitfalls

There are several common mistakes that students make that can be easily avoided.

✗ Lack of basic knowledge.
✗ Not checking current understanding.

✗ Use of medical jargon.
✗ Failure to deal with patient concerns.

Your ultimate aim is for the patient to take the medicine correctly. The way you communicate information to the patient and deal with concerns will affect compliance. Rates of non-compliance with medication vary from 8 to 95% with an average of 40–50%.

Compliance is likely to be poor for the following reasons.

1. Patient doesn't understand reason for taking medicines

Not taking treatment is the patient's right and unless the reason the medicine is prescribed has been understood, compliance is unlikely. Patients on warfarin for a DVT will see an improvement in symptoms after starting the drug but may see little point in continuing the medicine once they feel better. Patients with hypertension may not comply with antihypertensives since they do not feel unwell and do not appreciate the reason for being on them.

2. Regimen is complicated

Patients need to be very obsessional to obey a four-times-a-day drug regimen or cope with polypharmacy. Simple regimens and aids, such as drug cards, written instructions and dosset boxes, can help the patient take medication correctly.

3. Unpleasant side-effects

Some side-effects are inevitable, but patients are more likely to take their medicines if they understand the importance of the drug. In addition, if possible side-effects have been explained previously, patients are less likely to stop taking the medicine, as the effects will have been anticipated.

Checking prior knowledge is essential in this situation, since patients may have pre-existing concerns about warfarin. Patients are often aware that warfarin is the main constituent of rat poison. They may even mention it jokingly, as a cue that they are concerned about taking it. Do not laugh off their joke. Check whether it is a concern.

It is essential to stress the importance of continuing anticoagulant therapy long-term, and that medication should not be stopped without first discussing it with a doctor. Patients who feel well may not see the need to carry on taking their medicines, especially if they are more likely to bruise on it.

Example answer

Consultation	Commentary
Doctor: Hello Mrs. Jones. **Mrs. Jones:** Hello doctor. **Doctor:** I'm Doctor Wheatley. **Mrs. Jones:** Yes. I've seen you on the ward.	Introduces self.
Doctor: I see you've got your bags packed! **Mrs. Jones:** Yes! I'm going home today. **Doctor:** I'm glad to hear that. I've come to have a chat with you about your medicines.	Scene setting. Putting patient at ease.
Mrs. Jones: Oh good. They've made a few changes to my tablets so I could do with a chat about them.	Ascertaining prior knowledge.
Doctor: That's right. There have been some important changes to your tablets. How much do you understand about what's brought you back into hospital?	Reinforcing agenda. In this situation doctor and patient are similar. Checking prior knowledge.
Mrs. Jones: Well as you know I had my hip done a few weeks ago.	Allow dialogue.
Doctor: Yes.	Encouragement.
Mrs. Jones: I was coming along nicely but then I noticed a swelling in my calf. I thought nothing of it at first but it got worse and so I called my doctor.	
Doctor: I see.	Demonstrate listening.
Mrs. Jones: He sent me straight in here and they did an ultrasound of my leg.	
Doctor: And what did they say was going on?	Encourage dialogue and continue to ascertain patient understanding.

Mrs. Jones: They said I had a blood clot in my leg called a DVT.	
Doctor: That's right a deep vein thrombosis.	Reinforce patient knowledge.
Mrs. Jones: Yes, a deep vein thrombosis. So they started me on some blood-thinning tablets.	
Doctor: That's right. The medicine you have been started on is called warfarin. *(Pause)* I would like to spend a few minutes talking with you about the medicine since it's very important that it is taken properly at home.	Scene setting in context of patients understanding.

Stress importance of the conversation. |
Mrs. Jones: Okay doctor.	
Doctor: Warfarin belongs to the group of medicines known as anticoagulants. *(Pause)* It is used to prevent and treat the formation of harmful blood clots within the body.	Allow as many pauses as needed. Check patient body language to ensure they are following the consultation.
Mrs. Jones: Like my DVT.	
Doctor: Yes exactly. As you have discovered, a DVT can cause a painful swelling of the leg.	Relates to patient experience.
Mrs. Jones: Yes.	
Doctor: Sometimes the blood clot causing the DVT can travel to the lungs. This can make people breathless and sometimes very unwell indeed.	Identifying why compliance is important.

Also informing patient of risks of non-compliance. |
Mrs. Jones: Oh dear.	
Doctor: Fortunately, you are on the right blood-thinning medicine warfarin and you are already improving.	Reassurance and reinforcing current management plan.
Mrs. Jones: Yes, I'm feeling much better.	
Doctor: Even though you feel better it is very important that you carry on taking the warfarin for three months unless your doctor tells you to stop.	Notice that much of this is reinforcing the same information. Repeating important facts will assist patient understanding and retention of information.
Mrs. Jones: Three months?	

Doctor: Yes, 3 months. I know it sounds a long time but it is important not to stop the medicine unless told to.	Important to pick up on patient's cue to justify length of time for anticoagulation.
Mrs. Jones: I understand.	
Doctor: You will need regular blood tests to check that the warfarin is thinning your blood properly. *(pause)* Before you go I will arrange for you to be seen at the anticoagulant clinic next week.	Now we have outlined importance of compliance, proceed to discuss the monitoring of INR.
Mrs. Jones: Yes.	
Doctor: It is important to take the warfarin at the same time each day. The best time is early evening, around 6 pm.	Note use of short sentences. One point in each sentence.
Mrs. Jones: Okay.	
Doctor: You will go home with this monitoring book. It keeps a record of your blood tests. If your blood isn't thin enough, the doctors in the clinic will increase your dose of warfarin.	
Mrs. Jones: I see.	
Doctor: Is there anything you want to ask at this stage?	Keep checking the patient is following the discussion. Be prepared to re-explain and recap as often as required.
Mrs. Jones: No. I don't think so.	
Doctor: To recap. You will need regular blood tests at the anticoagulation clinic and will keep a record of your blood tests and warfarin dose in a monitoring book.	Recapping.
Mrs. Jones: Fine.	
Doctor: It is important that you do not take any new medicines without discussing with your doctor first.	New information. Stress importance.
Mrs. Jones: Oh!	
Doctor: Sometimes medicines, even herbal remedies bought over the counter, can alter how the warfarin works.	Pick up on cue and expand on information to clarify.
Mrs. Jones: I see.	

Doctor: It is especially important to avoid certain anti-inflammatory painkillers, such as ibuprofen and diclofenac. These can cause bleeding problems and should be avoided.	Essential safety information.
Mrs. Jones: Are there any side-effects I should be aware of?	Patients may not ask this so be prepared to mention it.
Doctor: Since warfarin prevents blood clots by thinning the blood, it also means that you may bruise more easily. If you cut yourself, you may notice that you take longer for the bleeding to stop.	You may wish to write the main points on a piece of paper for the patient, or go through the anticoagulant book with them.
Mrs. Jones: I see.	
Doctor: This is important if you are having an operation or dental work. The doctor will need to know you are taking warfarin.	
Mrs. Jones: Okay.	
Doctor: It is important not too drink too much alcohol whilst on warfarin. *(Pause)* Drinking in moderation is fine. Long-term heavy drinking or even binge drinking can have a dangerous effect on the way warfarin works.	Notice we only come to alcohol after covering the other essential information. Important to pick up on cues to see how this information is received.
Mrs. Jones: I see.	
Doctor: Do you have any questions about what I have been talking about?	
Mrs. Jones: No doctor.	
Doctor: Okay. Just to recap. You will need to take the warfarin for 3 months. *(Pause)* You will need regular blood tests at the clinic to monitor how thin your blood is. *(Pause)* You mustn't take any new medication without discussing it with your doctor.	Offer opportunity for further discussion. Summarise before finishing the consultation.
Mrs. Jones: Okay. Thank you doctor.	

We have included some fact sheets on the drugs that most frequently come up in the exam. The fact sheets are not exhaustive and we strongly recommend you cross-reference these sheets with the BNF. It is beyond the scope of this book to detail all aspects of taking different medicines. For example, preparations of the oral contraceptive pill vary and we advise reading around the subject to expand on the detail.

These scenarios are best prepared for by role-playing with colleagues. By doing this, you can get a feel for the sort of questions that patients may fire at you.

Fact sheet: Warfarin	
Facts you need to know	*Non-jargon ways to say it*
Indication • Oral anticoagulant in the treatment of venous thromboembolism	Warfarin belongs to the group of medicines known as *anticoagulants*. It is used to prevent and treat the formation of harmful blood clots within the body.
Mode of action • Vitamin K antagonist	Warfarin works by reducing the effects of vitamin K, which is a vitamin present in the body, essential in the process of blood-clotting.
How taken • Once daily in the evening	It is taken as a tablet once a day in the evening. It is important that you take it at the same time every day.
Side effects • Bruising and haemorrhage	Warfarin prevents blood clots forming by thinning the blood. If your blood is thinner, you are more likely to bruise if you knock yourself.
Monitoring • Check INR regularly	You will need a regular blood test to check that your blood is being thinned enough. It is very important that you have these blood tests, especially to make sure your blood doesn't get too thin.

Fact sheet: Warfarin—cont'd

Facts you need to know	Non-jargon ways to say it
• Anticoagulation card to record INR and dose of warfarin to be taken	You will be given a yellow booklet to record the dose and thinness of your blood. It is important to show this to your doctor when you have blood tests.
• Need to continue as long as advised	Your doctor will tell you how long you need to stay on the warfarin. You must not stop the warfarin on your own, as this could lead you to becoming unwell.

Hazards

• Drug–drug interactions	There are a few medicines that affect the way warfarin works. It is important that you do not take any new medicines without your doctor knowing. Even some over-the-counter medicines, including herbal remedies, can affect the way warfarin works.
• Increased risk of bleeding with non-steroidal anti-inflammatory drugs	Be very careful with painkillers such as aspirin or ibuprofen.
• Surgical procedures	Because warfarin thins the blood, you would be more likely to bleed after an operation. It is essential that you let doctors or dentists know you are taking warfarin if you ever need an operation or dental procedure.
• Alcohol	Alcohol in moderation is fine but binge drinking on warfarin can be very dangerous indeed.

Fact sheet: Warfarin drug–drug interactions

It is important to know which other drugs interact with warfarin. Many drugs can induce or inhibit the enzymes in the liver responsible for warfarin metabolism. Enzyme inducers will increase the livers ability to break down warfarin and thus decrease the INR. Enzyme inhibitors will lead to an increased INR and greater likelihood of bleeding.

Fact sheet: Warfarin drug–drug interactions—cont'd	
Enzyme inducers	*Enzyme inhibitors*
Phenytoin **C**arbamazepine **B**arbiturates **R**ifampicin **A**lcohol (chronic use) **G**riseofulvin **S**ulphonylureas	**O**meprazole **D**isulfiram **E**thanol (acute) **V**alproate **C**imetidine/ ciprofloxacin **E**rythromycin **S**ulphonamides
Mnemonic: **PCBRAGS**	Mnemonic: **ODEVICES**

Fact sheet: Corticosteroids	
Facts you need to know	*Non-jargon ways to say it*
Indication • Acute inflammatory conditions, auto-immune disorders, asthma	Steroid tablets work mainly by reducing inflammation. They are used to treat various conditions where inflammation occurs. For example: some auto-immune diseases; some types of muscle, skin, and joint diseases; asthma.
Mode of action • Anti-inflammatory	
How taken • Orally; best taken with food	
Side-effects • Osteoporosis (thinning of the bones) • Weight gain • Increased risk of infections • High blood pressure • Diabetes • Striae (purple marks on the skin) • Proximal myopathy (weakness in the leg muscles, especially when walking up stairs) • Mood swings	A short course of steroids usually causes no side-effects. Side-effects are more likely to occur if you take a long course of steroids (more than 2–3 months), or if you take short courses repeatedly.

Fact sheet: Steroids—cont'd	
Facts you need to know	*Non-jargon ways to say it*
Hazards • Adrenal suppression	Do not stop steroid tablets suddenly if you have been taking them for more than a few weeks. Sometimes you may need a short boost of steroid if your body is under strain from an infection or during an operation.
Monitoring	It is important that doctors looking after you know you are taking steroid tablets. Most people who take regular steroids carry a 'steroid card' and/or medic-alert bracelet. This details your dose of steroid and why you are taking it.

Fact sheet: Oral contraceptive pill	
Facts you need to know	*Non-jargon ways to say it*
Mode of action • Inhibits ovulation	The pill works mainly by changing the body's hormone balance so that you do not ovulate (you do not release an egg each month from your ovary).
• Mucus plugging	It causes the mucus made by the cervix to thicken and form a 'mucus plug' in the cervix. This makes it difficult for sperm to get through to the uterus (womb) to fertilise an egg.
• Thinning of uterine lining	It also makes the lining of the uterus thinner so that a fertilised egg will be less able to attach to the uterus.
How effective • 99% effective • Increased risk of pregnancy with poor compliance	It is over 99% effective if used correctly. This means that less than 1 woman in 100 using the pill correctly will become pregnant each year. Correct use means not missing any pills, and taking extra precautions when necessary.

Fact sheet: Oral contraceptive pill—cont'd	
Facts you need to know	*Non-jargon ways to say it*
Advantages • It is very effective • It does not interfere with sex • Periods are often lighter, less painful, and more regular	
How to take the pill • Take first pill on day one of period • Take pill at same time daily for 21 days • 7 day break followed by 21 days of pill again • If missed pill on day 1 need additional contraception for 21 days	Most brands of pill come in packs of 21. To start, take the first pill on the first day of your next period. You will be protected against pregnancy from then on. If you start the pill on any other day, you need an additional contraceptive method (such as condoms) for the first 7 days. Take your pill at about the same time each day for the 21 days.
Hazards • Drug–drug interactions including over the counter medicines, e.g. St Johns Wort	It is important to check with your doctor or pharmacist before starting any new medicines. This includes over the counter medicines. Otherwise there is a risk that you could become pregnant.
• Hypertension requiring 6-monthly blood pressure check-ups	The pill sometimes causes a rise in blood pressure. Therefore, if you take the pill you should have your blood pressure checked every 6 months.

PART 4

DISCUSSING TREATMENT ISSUES

10

Sexual issues

MALE SEXUAL DYSFUNCTION

Erectile dysfunction (the inability to achieve or maintain a penile erection sufficient for satisfactory sexual performance) is a common sexual problem, affecting half of men over age 40 at some point in their lives. It becomes more common with increasing age, yet only a small proportion of men seek help.

Mr. Clarke is a 48-year-old stockbroker. He has a past history of diabetes and was admitted to coronary care with chest pain six weeks ago. Serial ECGs and cardiac enzymes ruled out a myocardial infarction and he was discharged awaiting an exercise stress test.

He has made an appointment to discuss you prescribing him Viagra. He is happy to pay for a private prescription if necessary.

Essential skills required

- Professional, sensitive approach.
- Knowledge of causes of erectile dysfunction.
- Ability to discuss sexual issues without causing embarrassment.
- Awareness of exploring hidden agenda.

Think list

Your agenda
- Assess why he needs Viagra.
- Identify why he has erectile dysfunction.
- Explore psychological issues.
- Assess safety and appropriateness of prescribing Viagra.

Mr. Clarke's agenda
- Unease in discussing sexual problems.
- Used to being in control.
- May have undisclosed worries.
- Cardiac problems may be an issue.

Danger! Common pitfalls

This question is littered with hazards. Medical undergraduates find consultations regarding sexual matters difficult for several reasons:

✗ Personal embarrassment.
✗ Lack of exposure to sexual discussions during training.
✗ May find it amusing.
✗ It is a subject we tend to avoid in day-to-day consultations.
✗ Lack of personal knowledge.

Likewise Mr. Clarke will find it a difficult topic for reasons as follows:

✗ He may view erectile dysfunction as a poor reflection of his masculinity.
✗ He will not wish to discuss private matters with a stranger.
✗ Not used to discussing sexual matters.
✗ Lack of control.
✗ There may be undisclosed concerns he is reticent to discuss.

Pitfalls to avoid include:

✗ Unprofessional approach to patient.
✗ Not addressing hidden agenda.
✗ Not exploring cause of impotence.
✗ Inappropriate prescribing of Viagra.

Unprofessional approach to patient

You may be nervous about discussing sexual issues, but don't forget that Mr. Clarke is likely to be twice as nervous. A professional, unflappable approach will calm his nerves and instill confidence in you. Avoid at all costs using slang or joke terms. Even if the intention is to put the patient at ease it is more likely to backfire.

Doctor:	So Mr. Clarke. What seems to be the problem?
Mr. Clarke:	Well it's a bit embarrassing really.
Doctor:	Don't worry. I've heard it all before! Problem in the trouser department is it?
Mr. Clarke:	Well sort of.
Doctor:	Tool trouble is very common in men of your age. Lots of fellas have trouble getting it up.

This relaxed approach may suit some patients but can give the appearance of not taking the issue seriously. It is acceptable to use the same words as the patient but there are still some which should be avoided regardless.

Doctor: Hello Mr. Clarke. How can I help?
Mr. Clarke: Well it's a bit embarrassing really.
Doctor: That's okay. Take your time.
Mr. Clarke: I've been having trouble getting it up.
Doctor: I see.
Mr. Clarke: I was wondering if you could prescribe me Viagra.
Doctor: Well, I'd like to ask you a few more questions first if that's okay? How long have you had difficulty achieving an erection?

Not addressing hidden agenda

Doctor: Hello Mr. Clarke. How can I help you?
Mr. Clarke: I'd like some Viagra please.
Doctor: Certainly Mr. Clarke. Here's a prescription. Go home and enjoy yourself.

This approach may keep your consultations short but would be a definite fail in the exam! Around 10–15% of men with erectile dysfunction will have a psychological cause, and the remaining 85% will almost certainly have some emotional sequelae. A careful history should include asking whether the patient awakes with an early morning erection. If the patient awakes with an erection but is unable to achieve one during sexual arousal, a psychological cause is likely. Absence of morning erections suggests an underlying physiological cause.

The fact sheet below covers the more common psychological causes of erectile dysfunction. It is important to check for these. Impotence may be the first sign of depression or marital problems.

> **Fact sheet: Psychological causes of erectile dysfunction**
>
> - Depression
> - Anxiety
> - Guilt
> - Relationship difficulties
> - Work stress
> - Unresolved issues regarding own sexuality

In Mr. Clarke's case, let us not forget that he is under investigation for a heart problem.

- Is he worried that having sex may kill him?
- Has his admission to hospital caused him to question his place in the world?
- Has taking time off work affected him?
- How has his illness impacted on his relationship?

Not exploring cause of impotence

There is a physical cause for impotence in 85% of cases and these are listed in the fact sheet below.

> **Fact sheet: Physiological causes of erectile dysfunction**
>
> - Medicines
>   — This is a huge list, which is covered in the fact sheet on page 86.
> - Diabetes
>   — Vascular insufficiency
>   — Neuropathy
> - Vascular disease
> - Cancer related
>   — Radical prostatectomy
>   — Hormone manipulation
>   — Oestrogen—secreting tumours
> - Endocrine
>   — Low testosterone
>   — High oestrogen
> - Neurological disease
>   — Spinal cord injury
>   — Multiple sclerosis
>   — Parkinson's disease
> - Recreational substances
>   — Alcohol (brewer's droop)
>   — Nicotine
>   — Marijuana

Inappropriate prescribing of Viagra

Viagra or sildenafil, as it is generically known, is indicated for the treatment of erectile dysfunction. It is a potent and selective inhibitor of cGMP specific phosphodiesterase type 5 (PDE5).

In plain English, it blocks the breakdown of the compounds responsible for dilating the blood vessels, leading to an erection. Unfortunately, it also blocks the breakdown of nitrate-like medicines used for the treatment of angina (e.g. GTN, isosorbide), and giving Viagra to someone also taking a nitrate may cause a catastrophic sustained drop in blood pressure.

The other problem is that a bout of wild and crazy sex (especially if you haven't been able to do it for a while) is likely to take its toll if you have a heart condition. One needs to be clear that prescribing Viagra may cause more problems than it solves.

Example answer

Consultation	Commentary
Doctor: Mr. Clarke? **Mr. Clarke:** Yes? **Doctor:** Hello. My name is Dr. Stevens. **Mr. Clarke:** Bill Clarke. Pleased to meet you. **Doctor:** The practice nurse tells me you wanted to discuss your medicines with me. Is that correct?	Checks correct patient and introduces self.
Mr. Clarke: Yes, sort of. Well it's a bit embarrassing really. **Doctor:** That's okay. Take your time. **Mr. Clarke:** I've been having trouble getting it up.	Empathic unflappable approach.
Doctor: I see. **Mr. Clarke:** Well I was wondering whether you could prescribe me some Viagra. I'm happy to pay privately if necessary.	Encourage dialogue.

Doctor: Well before we talk about Viagra I'll need to ask you a few other questions, including your recent admission to hospital. Is that okay?	Acknowledge his objective of receiving Viagra and intent to return to that in a moment.
Mr. Clarke: Okay	
Doctor: How long have you had difficulty achieving an erection?	Professional terminology.
Mr. Clarke: About a month now. Maybe longer.	
Doctor: Go on.	Encourage dialogue.
Mr. Clarke: Well, I just don't seem to be able to get it up at all. My wife and I make love regularly but since coming back from hospital I haven't been able to.	Allow patient to give his own account. Note cue about hospital to follow up on.
Doctor: There are many possible reasons for this and to help work out why this has happened I'm afraid I need to ask some rather personal questions.	Acknowledge sensitive issue but explain why asking personal questions.
Mr. Clarke: Fine. No problem.	
Doctor: Does this problem happen just during lovemaking?	Specific questions to elicit if there is a physical or psychological cause.
Mr. Clarke: No, it's all the time.	
Doctor: Are you able to achieve an erection through masturbation?	
Mr. Clarke: To be honest, I don't think I've tried.	
Doctor: Do you still get early morning erections when you wake up?	
Mr. Clarke: No. I don't think I do.	
Doctor: You say, you've noticed this since your stay in hospital?	Suggests physical cause. Clarify previous cue.
Mr. Clarke: Yes.	
Doctor: The hospital has sent me a letter about your admission but it would be helpful to hear what happened from your viewpoint.	Encourage patient dialogue. Assess patients understanding, concerns, etc.
Mr. Clarke: Well, I was admitted with chest pain and spent a few days on coronary care. They had	

me on various drips, did lots of ECGs and loads of tests.

Doctor: And what did they say about the tests.

Checking knowledge.

Mr. Clarke: They said that I hadn't had a heart attack but they wanted to rule out angina. I'm due to have a treadmill test next week.

Doctor: It sounds like you've had a pretty stressful time.

Demonstrating empathy. Reflecting back to encourage further dialogue.

Mr. Clarke: It has been difficult and I'm off work until the treadmill test.

Doctor: Are you managing financially?

Is this adding to stress?

Mr. Clarke: Yes, that's not a problem. I'd just like to get back to normality.

Doctor: Sometimes after being in hospital, especially with chest pains, people worry whether making love may be harmful.

Explore fears. By referring to other peoples' experiences allows him to open up and realise his feelings are not unique.

Mr. Clarke: I suppose I was a bit worried, but the cardiac nurse said it would be fine.

Doctor: How are things with your wife?

Check impact of erectile dysfunction on relationship.

Mr. Clarke: They're fine. She's been really supportive and understanding. She tells me not to worry about it but I feel annoyed that I can't make love to her.

Doctor: It must be very frustrating.

Demonstrating empathy.

Mr. Clarke: It is. Very.

Doctor: I gather they altered your medicines whilst in hospital.

Returning to cues about hospital. Need to consider most likely physical cause.

Mr. Clarke: Yes. They started me on lots of new ones. Do you want to see the list?

(Hands list to doctor)

Doctor: So they started you on atenolol, isosorbide mononitrate and aspirin. Anything else?

Important since atenolol could be to blame and nitrates contraindicate Viagra.

Mr. Clarke: I was also given this GTN spray in case I got pain. I haven't used it though.	
Doctor: Because you haven't had pain or haven't wanted to take it?	Clarify. Check whether he has been getting pain.
Mr. Clarke: Because I've had no pain.	
Doctor: I'm glad to hear it. Are you taking any other medicines?	
Mr. Clarke: Just the gliclazide for my diabetes.	
Doctor: Lets just talk about what may be going on here. It is very common for men at some point in life to have difficulty in getting an erection. *(Pause)* Before we talk about Viagra we need to address possible causes of erectile dysfunction. *(Pause)* With all you have been through in the past 2 months, there are quite a few reasons why this may be happening.	Reassuring approach. Lots of pauses to allow for response. Also breaks up talking. Time for questions. Check he is following.
Mr. Clarke: Okay.	
Doctor: It is possible that one of the medicines you have been started on may be responsible for this. Around 15% of men started on atenolol experience erectile difficulties.	
Mr. Clarke: Can I stop taking it then?	
Doctor: I wouldn't advise stopping it without discussion with the cardiologists. I will contact them and ask their advice as to an alternative heart medicine. I suspect they will want to see the results of the treadmill test before making a decision.	Advise safest plan. Inform him of the plan but give him realistic time frame.
Mr. Clarke: Okay.	
Doctor: The other issue is whether we should give you Viagra. *(Pause)* Viagra can work well in some people but there are certain medicines it reacts with. You are on such a	Now onto the reason he has come to see you. Patient needs to understand why you will not prescribe Viagra.

medicine and if you took Viagra you would become very unwell.

Mr. Clarke: Really?

Doctor: Absolutely. If you took Viagra it could have drastic consequences. You would become seriously unwell.

Need to reinforce this several times if necessary.

Mr. Clarke: Oh. I don't mind paying for it myself.

Doctor: I promise you it has nothing to do with cost. It is to do with your health. *(Pause)* What we need to do is wait for this treadmill test and then see what the cardiologists suggest about your medicines. *(Pause)* I suspect that this may be due to your medicines and we should deal with this side of things first before considering other causes.

Reinforce again and reiterate plan to tackle the erectile dysfunction.

Mr. Clarke: Okay.

Doctor: There are many causes for erectile dysfunction. The most likely cause for you is related to your medicines. However, it is very common for men to experience this after a period of upset or stress. With all you've been through in the past couple of months I think we should at least consider that this might be a factor.

Summarise most likely cause but lay down tentative foundations to explore psychological issues at a future session.

Mr. Clarke: That sounds reasonable. What happens now?

Doctor: I will contact the cardiologists and discuss your medicines with them. I suggest we make an appointment to see you in two weeks to see what they recommend and discuss the results of the treadmill test.

Reiterate the plan and arrange follow-up.

Mr. Clarke: Okay.

Doctor: I know it must be frustrating to wait another couple of weeks but whatever you do, don't alter your medicines. Also don't be tempted to buy any Viagra on the internet. It really would be dangerous for you.

Empathy and revisit safety aspects.

Mr. Clarke: Okay doctor. **Doctor:** Is there anything else you would like to discuss at the moment? *(Mr. Clarke shakes his head)* Well I'll see you in 2 weeks time.	Opportunity for further questions.

Obviously you will need to be flexible in your consultation. The history of not experiencing early morning erections strongly suggests a physical cause for erectile dysfunction, and the time frame coincides with starting the β-blocker. In the absence of drug causes (see fact sheet below), it would be important to explore whether diabetes was a factor.

Even though 85% of erectile dysfunction cases are due to physical causes, it is important to explore psychological causes. In addition, a good candidate will assess what effect the erectile dysfunction is having on the man and relationships.

The examiners are looking for a professional empathic approach. You need to demonstrate that you are comfortable discussing intimate and sometimes embarrassing issues with patients.

Fact sheet: Drugs causing erectile dysfunction

- Antidepressants
  - Tricyclics
  - MAOIs
  - SSRIs
- Antihypertensives
  - β-blockers
  - Methyldopa
  - Prazosin
- Gastroprotectants
  - Cimetidine
  - Omeprazole
- Diuretics
  - Thiazides
  - Spironolactone
- Antiandrogens
  - Finasteride
- Anticholinergics
- Digoxin
- Antiepileptics
  - Carbamazepine
  - Gabapentin
  - Phenytoin

TAKING A SEXUAL HISTORY

Candidates often find talking about sexual issues difficult. Many reasons for this are outlined in this chapter. It is less likely that you will get a scenario that focuses solely on taking a sexual history. It is more likely that you will be given a consultation that requires you at some point to address sexual issues. A sexual history may need to be taken whilst discussing the following:

- contraception
- erectile dysfunction
- termination of pregnancy
- HIV testing
- sexually transmitted infections
- carcinoma of the cervix
- pyrexia of unknown origin
- hepatitis.

Essential skills required

- Professional approach.
- Ability to take a sexual history.

Danger! Common pitfalls

- ✗ Being judgemental.
- ✗ Making assumptions.
- ✗ Inappropriate use of slang.
- ✗ Not contextualising questions.

Being judgemental

A person's sexual attitudes and conduct will depend upon many things, including:

- religious and spiritual beliefs
- social attitudes
- past experiences
- media
- self image.

What is normal sexual practice for you may be considered obscene to someone else. Likewise, a patient may consider what they do to be normal, whilst you view it as immoral. The important thing is to be unshockable and non-judgemental. You should not judge a fat person for having a heart attack or a smoker for having a stroke. Likewise, you should not judge a person according to their sexual conduct (unless it breaks the law).

Making assumptions

This once again illustrates the importance of checking prior knowledge, in this case your knowledge. Do not assume anything. For example, a patient who presents requesting an HIV test may do so for a number of reasons. Making assumptions could have a disastrous effect on the consultation.

Doctor:	Hello Mr. Clarke. How can I help you?
Mr. Clarke:	I was wondering if I could have an HIV test please.
Doctor:	Certainly Mr. Clarke but first I'd like to ask you how many unprotected homosexual contacts you have had in the past year. *(Mr. Clarke reaches across the desk and punches the doctor)*

Checking the reason for this request may make things clearer and less likely to offend.

Doctor:	Hello Mr. Clarke. How can I help you?
Mr. Clarke:	I was wondering if I could have an HIV test please.
Doctor:	Of course. Is there a particular reason that you feel you need to have an HIV test?
Mr. Clarke:	Yes. I am immigrating to Australia and am required to provide evidence of a negative HIV test.

Inappropriate use of slang

Patients are understandably nervous about discussing sexual issues, and use of stilted words can make the consultation embarrassingly painful. Appropriate use of slang can relax the patient and make them feel that you are empathic and human. However, over zealous use of slang is offensive and may destroy the professional relationship.

Not contextualising questions

As doctors, we are given the privilege of being able to ask patients some of their most intimate secrets, things they may not even tell their loved ones. This is even more likely when discussing sexual issues. Patients will be comfortable answering intimate questions only if they can understand your reason for asking. Otherwise it may appear to be perverted voyeurism.

Doctor:	Hello Mr. Clarke. How can I help you?
Mr. Clarke:	I was wondering if I could have an HIV test please. I'm concerned I may be HIV-positive.
Doctor:	Have you had unprotected anal sex recently?
Mr. Clarke:	I beg your pardon!

Although it is reasonable for the doctor to ask searching questions to give an indication of Mr. Clarke's risk of exposure to HIV, the above question is too direct, and sprung upon him without warning. It is important to check about high-risk behaviour, but the patient needs to understand the reason for such questions.

Doctor:	Hello Mr. Clarke. How can I help you?
Mr. Clarke:	I was wondering if I could have an HIV test please. I'm concerned I may be HIV-positive.
Doctor:	What I'd first like to do is ask you some questions which relate to risk factors to exposure to HIV. Some of them will be questions about your sex life.
Mr. Clarke:	That's fine doctor.

Incidentally, HIV testing is covered later in the book.

General Points

- Use clear unambiguous open-ended questions.
- Start with a general non-threatening question.

- When discussing sexual behaviour, use words like 'how', 'what' and 'where'. Do not use 'why' as it may appear judgemental.
- Once a rapport is established, do not be afraid to ask direct questions.
- Questions about sexual partners are important since they may be at risk of sexually transmitted infections (STIs).
- Asking about knowledge and use of condoms provides an opportunity for further information and education.

In the fact sheet below we have provided a checklist of headings that are relevant to a sexual history. Familiarise yourself with the main points and be prepared to adapt them as part of other consultations.

Fact sheet: Checklist of headings relevant to a sexual history	
Checklist	*Clinical relevance*
Physical symptoms • Nature of the problem • Time course • Any general sexual concerns	Vital information in order to make a differential diagnosis Patient-centred approach
Previous diagnosis of STIs • Previous sexual health issues • Knowledge of increased risk • Vaccinations, e.g. hepatitis • Symptoms and diagnoses of recent sexual partners	Previous health issues do not always go away, e.g. herpes; likewise HIV or hepatitis B and C related disease might be ongoing Risk of catching whatever the partner had if it is transmissible
Sexual behaviour • Regular/ casual sexual contact • Last sexual contact • Type of sexual contact with each partner • Condom use • Erectile dysfunction • Sexual contact with people from overseas • Non-consensual sex	Important to identify high-risk behaviour and their extent. STIs are more likely to be transmitted by certain high-risk practices and consistent condom use will minimise this Certain countries have a huge prevalence of HIV and sexual contact with someone from a high-risk area increases the chance of transmission
Relationship history • Regular partner • Partners sexual activity • Casual partners	Even someone with only one sexual partner is at risk of STIs if their partner practices high-risk behaviour

Fact sheet: Checklist of headings relevant to a sexual history—cont'd	
Checklist	*Clinical relevance*
Females • Menstrual cycle • Contraception • Cervical screening history • Obstetric history including terminations	Essential information in any female sexual health history
Drug and alcohol use • Patterns and frequency of use • Injecting drug use • Harm minimisation strategies	This is not just to identify HIV risk from injections. People who get drunk or high are more likely to have casual sexual contacts. In addition these people are at greater risk of non-consensual sex
Medication • Current medications • Known drug allergies	Essential to know in any history and may give clues to previous sexual issues

URETHRAL DISCHARGE

Mr. Adams is a 29-year-old businessman presenting with a urethral discharge. Take a focussed history from him.

Essential skills required

- Knowledge of causes of urethral discharge and ability to differentiate between them.
- Ability to obtain relevant information.
- Professional approach.
- Ability to take relevant sexual history.

Think list

Your agenda	*Mr. Adams' agenda*
• Obtain clear focussed history. • Formulate a differential . diagnosis • Address any questions or anxieties.	• Concerned that it is a sexually transmitted disease. • Issues regarding his wife finding out that he has been having an affair.

Danger! Common pitfalls

There are several common mistakes that students make that can be easily avoided.

✗ Lack of basic knowledge.
✗ Not checking current understanding and concerns.
✗ Assuming cause is infective.
✗ Not acknowledging his concerns.

Assuming cause is infective

Although the most common causes of urethral discharge are infective, there are some that are not. There will be times that the patient has not had a sexual encounter leading to the symptoms, and proceeding straight away with a sexual history may be inappropriate.

Sometimes a patient will present with reticence, having had a sexual encounter with someone other than a regular partner. The patient will be naturally worried about the implications to the relationship and the partner's health. Sometimes the presentation will be the first thing that suggests his or her partner has been having sex with someone else. Do not assume anything. Be open minded, unshockable and non-judgemental.

Fact sheet: Causes of urethritis	
Common causes	*Neisseria gonorrhoea* *Chlamydia trachomatis* *Mycoplasma* spp
Uncommon causes	Herpes simplex *Candida albicans* Human papilloma virus
Non-infectious causes	Trauma Chemical irritants Carcinoma

Fact sheet: Causes of urethral discharge	
Essential questions	*Clinical relevance*
• How long after sex did it start?	24–72 hours after suggests gonococcus Non-gonococcal urethritis is more indolent
• What colour is the discharge and how much?	Gonococcal discharge is usually purulent, whilst non-gonococcal is thin and colourless
• Does it hurt to pass water?	Dysuria is frequent in urethritis but in the absence of urethral discharge suggests a UTI
• Have you noticed any blood when you pass water?	Haematuria is uncommon in urethritis and suggests urinary tract disease
• Is it painful when you open your bowels or when you sit down?	Pain in the penis or perineum on defecation suggests prostatitis
• Is there any pain in your testicles?	Suggests epididymo-orchitis
• Have you had any fevers, chills, sweats or shakes? Any pain anywhere?	Systemic symptoms such as rigors, fever or loin pain suggests a bacterial UTI
• Any joint pains or rashes?	Pustular rash and arthralgia with fever suggest disseminated gonorrhoea Reiter's syndrome follows urethritis and includes arthritis, conjunctivitis, circinate balanitis and keratoderma blenorrhagica
• Full sexual history including past partners needs to be taken (see p. 87).	Relevant with regards contact tracing, identifying at risk behaviour, etc.

HIV TESTING

Jane Williams is a 30-year-old woman. She attends surgery requesting an HIV test. How would you deal with this request?

Essential skills required

- Knowledge of HIV infection and testing.
- Sensitive sympathetic approach.
- Understanding of ethical issues concerning HIV testing.
- Anticipate and manage Ms. Williams' concerns.

Think list

Your agenda	*Ms. Williams' agenda*
• Obtain clear focussed history.	• Worried she has HIV.
• Assess whether high risk of HIV exposure.	• May not understand difference between HIV and AIDS.
• Give effective pre-test counselling.	• Concerns about implications of a positive test.
• Ensure follow-up for result.	

Danger! Common pitfalls

There are several common mistakes that students make that can be easily avoided.

✗ Lack of basic knowledge.

✗ Not checking current understanding and concerns.

✗ Use of medical jargon.

✗ Not acknowledging her concerns.

A few years ago, trained counsellors were the only ones to do the pre-test HIV counselling. It is becoming more common for non-specialist doctors to be required to do this. Although it is unlikely that you will be expected to fully counsel someone in the exam, we have included a checklist of relevant points on this topic for completeness. We have known of students to be quizzed on things they may discuss with a patient requesting a test.

This consultation may involve educating the patient about HIV and AIDS, as well as discussing behavioural aspects such as safe sex.

Fact sheet: Counselling for an HIV test	
	Important points to explore
Take STD history	• Determine HIV risk • Determine when exposure to risk occurred
Previous HIV test	• Check date and result
Explanation of test	• Rationale for testing (early detection can improve long-term prognosis and reduce risk of transmission)

Fact sheet: Counselling for an HIV test—cont'd	
	Important points to explore
	• HIV antibody test • Difference between HIV and AIDS • 3-month 'window period' from exposure to development of antibodies • Advise if repeat test will be necessary • Confidentiality issues around HIV testing should be discussed. Patients should be advised about protecting their own confidentiality by carefully considering and limiting whom they tell • Obtain informed consent from patient • It is recommended that all HIV results are given in person by medical practitioners
Implications of a negative result	• Provides reassurance • Provides opportunity to discuss prevention through safe sex • If exposure to risk was less than 3 months ago, a repeat test may be indicated
Implications of a confirmed positive result	• Discuss the difference between HIV and AIDS • Check if there is a trusted support person available • Discuss medical follow-up and treatments • Support lifestyle changes, e.g. diet, smoking, rest, safe sex • Contact tracing of past sexual partners

Fact sheet: Legal and social consequences of testing positive for HIV
• When applying for a mortgage, people can be asked whether they have ever had an HIV test. If they admit to it they may be refused cover. The exception to this is if the test was a mandatory test for insurance. • HIV status is enquired about at employment medicals. Patients are not legally obliged to divulge this information. • If tested positive the patient will be strongly encouraged to consent to their GP and dentist being notified. This will be entered on their permanent records. • If tested positive, the patient's partner(s) should be informed.

Needle stick injury

The other scenario that may come up in the exam concerns the management of a needle stick injury.

Miss Gill Freeman is a 24-year-old staff nurse. She presents to accident and emergency having had a needle stick injury from a known HIV-positive patient.

In this situation you must maintain a calm manner as the healthcare professional will be terrified that she will become HIV-positive. Time is important here and you need to act quickly if post-exposure prophylaxis is to be effective. For this reason closed directive questions are required early on in the consultation. We would suggest something like this:

Doctor:	I understand this must all be rather distressing for you. It is important that we deal with this as quickly as possible and if necessary start you on some appropriate treatment. Before we do that I need to ask you a few important questions. Is that okay?
Miss Freeman:	Yes, that's fine.
Doctor:	If I interrupt you at any point, I'm not doing it to be rude. It's just important that we get a few vital details quickly and then go from there.

This will allow you to make a rapid assessment of level of risk so that you can develop a treatment plan and arrange appropriate support/counselling.

Fact sheet: Assessment in needle stick injury	
Essential questions	*Clinical relevance*
When did the needle stick injury occur?	Timing is important, as post exposure prophylaxis should be given as soon as possible
Do you know what sort of needle it was?	Transmission risk is greater with a large bore hollow needle
Had the needle come into direct contact with the patient's blood?	Greater risk if there is evidence that the needle was in direct contact with the patient's blood

Fact sheet: Assessment in needle stick injury—cont'd	
Essential questions	*Clinical relevance*
How deep was the injury?	Transmission more likely with deep injury
What did you do afterwards?	Risk of transmission lessened by patient making injury bleed afterwards and washing area thoroughly in hot soapy water
Do you have details about the patient or where we can get access to their details?	Important to find out information about the 'donor' patient including: • HIV viral load • stage of disease • current medication and previous medication history • hepatitis B and C status

If considered a high-risk exposure, the colleague will be started immediately on prophylaxis. She will need to be tested for HIV at appropriate times and will require pre-test counselling for this. This should include discussions about other risk factors for HIV, and discussions about sexual partners who may be at risk, should she seroconvert to HIV.

DISCUSSING A VASECTOMY WITH A MALE PATIENT

Mr. Brannigan is married with four children. He has requested an appointment to discuss having a vasectomy.

Essential skills required

- Knowledge about vasectomy.
- Sensitive professional approach.
- Anticipate and manage Mr. Farmer's concerns and questions.

Think list

Your agenda
- Check he is certain that he wants a vasectomy.
- Discuss procedure for vasectomy.

Mr. Brannigan's agenda
- May be embarrassed.
- May have concerns about the operation.

- Address any questions or anxieties.

- May have been pressured to have the vasectomy.

Danger! Common pitfalls

There are several common mistakes that students make that can be easily avoided.

✘ Lack of basic knowledge.
✘ Not checking current understanding and reasons for request.
✘ Use of medical jargon.
✘ Not acknowledging his concerns.

Basically this consultation has two parts:

- *First part*—explore why he is requesting a vasectomy and ensure this is an appropriate decision.
- *Second part*—impart information about the procedure and enable patient to come to an informed decision.

First part—information to explore

Why does he want a vasectomy?

- It is important that he is certain that he wants this operation since it is irreversible.
- Does he have children and is there any chance he may want more in the future?
- Was this his decision, his partners or both?

What has lead to this decision at this point in time?

- It is important that a decision such as this has been reached over time and not rushed.
- It is not wise to make such a decision at time of crisis or change, especially after a new baby or termination of pregnancy.
- It is important not to make this decision if there are any major problems between the patient and partner. It will not solve any sexual problems.

What are his partner's views?

- It is better to have both partner and patient present to discuss issues.
- If the partner is not present, explore why.

- It is not a legal requirement to get the partner's permission but it is less likely to be a wise plan if only one of the couple wants the vasectomy to occur.

Second part—impart information

Fact sheet: Vasectomy	
Facts you need to know	*Non-jargon ways to say it*
What it is? • Operation to cut the vas deferens, preventing sperm access to semen	• Vasectomy is a small operation to cut the vas deferens. • This is the tube that takes sperm from the testes to the penis. • Sperm are made in the testes. Once the vas deferens is cut, sperm can no longer get into the semen that is ejaculated during sex.
How reliable? • Very reliable; 1 in 1000 procedures unsuccessful	• Vasectomy is very reliable—but not quite 100%. • 1 in 1000 vasectomies is unsuccessful and shows sperm in the semen after the operation.
What does it involve? • Usually done under local anaesthetic • Dissolvable stitches • Takes about 15 minutes • Advise to wear tight fitting pants and avoid lifting for a week	• It is usually done with a local anaesthetic (but is sometimes done under a general anaesthetic). • Local anaesthetic is injected into a small area of skin on either side of the scrotum above the testes. • A small cut is then made to these numbed areas of skin. • The vas deferens can be seen quite easily under the cut skin. It is cut, and the two ends are tied. • There is usually some discomfort and bruising for a few days afterwards. • Wearing tight fitting underpants day and night for a week after the operation can help it. • It is also best not to do heavy work, exercise, or lifting for a week or so after the operation.

Fact sheet: Vasectomy—cont'd	
Facts you need to know	*Non-jargon ways to say it*
Advantages • It is permanent • More effective, than female sterilisation	• It is permanent and you don't have to think of contraception again. • It is easier to do, and more effective, than female sterilisation.
Risks • Bruising • Post-operative pain	• There is likely to be bruising around the operation site but this will go after a week or so. • A small number of men have a dull ache in the scrotum for a few months after the operation.
Sex issues • Sex as soon as comfortable • Alternative contraception required until two sperm-free samples produced	• You can resume sex as soon as it is comfortable to do so. • You will have to use other methods of contraception (such as condoms) until you provide two semen specimens that are clear of sperm. • Some sperm will survive 'upstream' from the cut vas deferens for a few weeks. • You must wait till the 'all clear' before stopping other forms of contraception.

11

Epilepsy and driving

Mr. Peter Adams is a 42-year-old long-distance lorry driver. He was seen in casualty having had a possible fit and was discharged home pending further investigations. His brain CT is normal but the EEG confirms a diagnosis of epilepsy.

He has attended outpatients for the results. Discuss the diagnosis and its implications for driving.

Essential skills required

- Generic breaking bad news skills.
- Knowledge of legal aspects of driving following an epileptic seizure.
- Ability to manage angry patient.

Think list

Your objectives	Mr. Adams' view
• To give Mr. Adams the diagnosis.	• Feels a lot of fuss made over nothing.
• Inform him of legalities of driving (see fact sheet, p. 103).	• Angry with diagnosis.
	• Driving is essential for his job.

Danger! Common pitfalls

There are several common mistakes that students make that can be easily avoided.

- ✗ Not checking current understanding.
- ✗ Lack of basic knowledge.
- ✗ Use of medical jargon.
- ✗ Inappropriate response to angry patient.

In some ways this consultation is no different to a breaking bad news scenario. We often forget that breaking bad news is not limited to telling patients that they are dying or have cancer. It is whenever you give someone information they do not want to hear. Often by forgetting this, we give the distressing information too quickly, resulting in a shell-shocked and distressed individual.

The problem with this particular scenario is that candidates feel the need to rush the breaking bad news part in order to get to the driving bit. Rushing the first part will make the second part of the consultation much harder.

Once you have given the Mr. Adams the diagnosis you need to broach the subject of driving. The rules for fitness to drive are complex, and there are major differences between the rules for group 1 and group 2 drivers.

- Group 1 drivers: motor cars and motor cycles.
- Group 2 drivers: lorries and buses.

Patients with epilepsy must not drive a car for 1 year after a daytime fit. In addition, Mr. Adams is a group 2 driver and legally must not drive a lorry for 10 years after a fit.

This news will have a huge impact on Mr. Adams since his job depends on him being able to drive a lorry. He is likely to be angry, shocked and quite likely not to believe you. Often patients will suggest that you have got the wrong diagnosis and try to convince you not to label them as having epilepsy.

Let us not forget what your role is here.

1. You are to advise Mr. Adams that he has epilepsy.
2. You are to advise Mr. Adams that he should inform the DVLA of his diagnosis.

It is not your decision whether he should drive or not. The decision rests with the DVLA. You can inform him of the DVLA guidelines and that he should not drive until he has been in contact with them.

The reason students find this scenario difficult is because they get embroiled in the complexities of Mr. Adams' inevitable response. You have basically told him he cannot do his job any more. He isn't going to take this lying down! Expect some of the following responses:

'You've got the wrong diagnosis. The tests are wrong'

'I didn't really pass out. I remember being conscious all the time.'

'Please don't put this in my notes. Please don't tell anyone I had a fit. I'm begging. My life depends on this job.'

'Sod you. I don't care what you say. I'm not going to tell the DVLA.'

The DVLA give clear guidelines for doctors and their role in advising patients who may have a condition that may affect their driving.

- Inform patients that they have a legal duty to inform the DVLA.
- If the patient refuses to accept the diagnosis, suggest that the patient seek a second opinion. Offer to make appropriate arrangements for the patient to do so. You should advise the patient not to drive until the second opinion has been obtained.
- If the patient continues to drive, make every effort to convince them not to. With the patient's permission you could talk with relatives to help convince the patient.
- If a patient continues to drive against advice, you should disclose relevant medical information immediately, in confidence, to the medical adviser at DVLA.
- Before you inform the DVLA you should inform the patient of your decision to do so. Once you have informed the DVLA you should inform the patient in writing that the disclosure has been made.

Fact sheet: Guidelines for driving with medical conditions

Patients with epilepsy should not drive a motorcar for 1 year after a daytime fit. They must also not drive for a year after a nocturnal fit, unless they have had an attack whilst asleep more than 3 years ago and have not had any awake attacks since that sleep attack. Patients with epilepsy may not drive a lorry or a bus for 10 years after any epileptic attack. For such patients to regain their licence they must have not required any medication to treat their epilepsy for 10 years and be deemed to 'not be a source of danger whilst driving'.

Condition	Group 1	Group 2
• Angina	Driving must cease when symptoms occur at rest or at the wheel. DVLA need not be notified	If continuing symptoms, licence revoked
• Angioplasty	No driving for 1 week	No driving for 6 weeks
• Myocardial infarction	No driving for at least 4 weeks	No driving for at least 6 weeks
• CABG	No driving for at least 4 weeks	No driving for at least 6 weeks
• Pacemaker implant	No driving for 1 week	No driving for at least 6 weeks
• First seizure	One year off driving with medical review before restarting driving	Following a first unprovoked seizure, drivers must demonstrate ten years freedom from further seizures, without anticonvulsant medication in that time

The reader is advised to consult the document 'At a glance guide to the current standards of fitness to drive, DVLA, Swansea, UK, 2001'. This document gives full details of the fitness-to-drive rules. These rules are lengthy and complex and beyond the scope of this text.

12

Discussing dialysis with a patient

Miss Jackson is 26 years old and works as a personal assistant in a large law firm. She has been under the nephrologists for 6 years with glomerulonephritis. Despite being compliant with her medicines, her renal function has continued to deteriorate and it is anticipated that she will need to start renal replacement therapy (dialysis) in the next 6 months.

This was discussed with her by one of your colleagues at the last appointment and you have been asked to see her to discuss dialysis options.

Essential skills required

- Knowledge of dialysis and options available (see fact sheet, p. 109).
- Ability to discuss complex issues in a clear concise way.
- Use of non-medical jargon.
- Anticipate and address patient's concerns.

Think list

Your objectives
- Explain need for dialysis and options available.
- Ensure patient compliance.
- Discuss pros and cons of different dialysis options.
- Explain follow-up plans.

Miss Jackson's view
- May not have understood that she needs dialysis.
- Concerns of how dialysis will impact on lifestyle.
- Concerns how starting dialysis will affect her appearance.

Danger! Common pitfalls

There are several common mistakes that students make that can be easily avoided.

✗ Lack of basic knowledge.
✗ Not checking current understanding.

✗ Use of medical jargon.
✗ Failure to deal with patient concerns.
✗ Lack of basic knowledge.

It is impossible to counsel a patient about the issues concerning dialysis unless you have a working understanding of the subject. We strongly advise you to revise the essentials of renal medicine as covered in *Final MB: A Guide for Success in Clinical Medicine*. It covers the basic principles of managing renal failure and the different dialysis options available to patients. A candidate that clearly has no understanding of the subject will not instil any confidence in a nervous patient.

Not checking current understanding

Do not assume that the patient understands the purpose of today's consultation. Even if your colleague has documented that they have discussed the need for dialysis last time, this does not mean the patient retained all this information. Starting the consultation without checking current understanding could be disastrous.

Doctor:	Hello Miss Jackson. I'm Dr. Abraham. I'm here to discuss dialysis options with you.
Miss Jackson:	I beg your pardon?
Doctor:	Well as you know, you renal disease has progressed so much that we now need to put you on dialysis and as Dr. Chambers mentioned last time we need to talk about options.
Miss Jackson:	I don't know what you're talking about.
Doctor:	Yes you do. Dr. Chambers talked to you about it last time.
Miss Jackson:	No one has mentioned this before! What do you mean my kidneys aren't working?

There is very little chance of salvaging this consultation now, since the patient has just received devastating news and will not be able to handle any further information. By the end of this book you will be sick of us reminding you to check prior knowledge, but hopefully it will prevent you having to deal with the consequences of such a basic mistake.

Doctor:	Hello Miss Jackson.
Miss Jackson:	Hello doctor.
Doctor:	I'm Dr. Abraham. We haven't met before.
Miss Jackson:	No. Last time I saw Dr. Chambers.
Doctor:	Since it's the first time we've met, would you mind giving me a brief outline of what you understand has been happening with your health recently.
Miss Jackson:	Well, I know that my kidneys are not working as well.
Doctor:	That's right. Did Dr. Chambers say anything about what we need to do about this?
Miss Jackson:	I know he said something but can't quite remember what he said.
Doctor:	Would you like me to explain a little about it now?
Miss Jackson:	Yes please.

From here you can re-explain the issues of renal failure and dialysis. Don't forget that the principles are the same as breaking bad news. Fire a warning shot, explaining as much as the patient wants to hear.

Use of medical jargon

Doctor:	As you know, your IgA glomerulonephritis is progressive and resistant to immunosuppression. We therefore need to explore renal replacement therapy options. Your choices are haemo or CAPD. I'll explain a bit about them in a minute.

Failure to deal with patient concerns

For a young patient to contemplate long-term dialysis is a major lifestyle change. Any form of dialysis relies on strict patient compliance or else things can go disastrously wrong.

Your priority may differ greatly from hers. Continuous ambulatory peritoneal dialysis may afford patients a degree of freedom but could be completely unacceptable cosmetically. (If you didn't understand the last sentence, you can't have read the renal chapter from 'Final MB'. Go and read up on it now!).

Doctor:	CAPD is straightforward and gives you freedom.
Miss Jackson:	I'm not having CAPD. How can I wear a bikini if I've got a tube sticking in my belly?
Doctor:	There are more important things at stake here than wearing a bikini.
Miss Jackson:	I don't care! I'm not having it.

It is often better to acknowledge concerns, identify their importance and promise to address them either now or at a later point.

Doctor:	CAPD is straightforward and gives you freedom.
Miss Jackson:	I'm not having CAPD. How can I wear a bikini if I've got a tube sticking in my belly?
Doctor:	That's obviously very important to you.
Miss Jackson:	Absolutely.
Doctor:	That's why it is so important for us to discuss the different treatments so we can find the one that is best suited for you. *(Pause)* There are pros and cons to each of the treatments. It is important to consider that it is very important to have dialysis to prevent you becoming unwell. Sometimes we have to compromise a little to get the best option for you.
Miss Jackson:	I see.

Fact sheet: Issues to consider in planning dialysis	
Haemodialysis	*Continuous ambulatory peritoneal dialysis (CAPD)*
• Requires access via central line or arterio-venous fistula • Need to come into hospital at least three times a week for dialysis • Will need to plan job around fixed dialysis sessions • Limited training required • Harder (but not impossible) to arrange holidays • Strict fluid balance required between dialysis sessions • Very efficient at removing toxins • Patients tend to have a better nutritional status • Lower incidence of complications • Contraindicated in severe ischaemic heart disease	• Access via Tenchkoff catheter • No need to come into hospital • More flexibility with work. Can be integrated into most jobs • Patients require extensive training • More freedom in holidays • Patients can regulate their fluid balance via choice of CAPD bags • Less efficient • Poorer nutritional status due to loss of proteins via dialysate bags • Peritonitis is a possible complication • Caution in chronic lung disease

PART 5

TAKING A FOCUSSED HISTORY

13

Anaemia

A 45-year-old woman is referred to the gastroenterology clinic by her GP. The referral letter is as follows:

Dear Dr.

I would be grateful if you would see and investigate Mrs. Tinker who presents with anaemia. This was discovered by the blood transfusion service when she attended to give blood. She regularly gives blood and has not been refused before by the transfusion service.

Yours faithfully

Dr. N. Hamad
General Practitioner

NB blood results were as follows:

Hb	8.5 g/dl	(11.5–15.0 g/dl)
MCV	65 fl	(80–95 fl)
Serum iron	5.0 micromol/l	(8.8–27.0 micromol/l)
Transferrin	4.1 g/l	(2.0–3.2 g/l)
Iron saturation	15.2%	(14.0–55.0%)

Please take a structured history from this patient to determine a differential diagnosis for the cause of her anaemia. Explain to the patient what investigations she requires and why.

Essential skills required

- Professional, sensitive approach.
- Knowledge of differential diagnosis of anaemia (fact sheet, p. 121).
- Knowledge of how to investigate iron deficiency anaemia (fact sheet, p. 123).
- Awareness of exploring hidden agenda.

Think list

Your agenda	Mrs. Tinker's agenda
• Take a clear focussed history.	• She doesn't know why she is anaemic.
• Formulate a differential diagnosis.	
• Pick up on cues from Mrs. Tinker.	• She may be unsure why she has been referred to a gastroenterologist.
• Explain plan of action.	

Danger! Common pitfalls

✗ Lack of knowledge of differential diagnosis and presentation of anaemia.

✗ Failure to pick up on Mrs. Tinker's agenda.

✗ Failure to address concerns and respond to cues.

This patient has an iron deficiency anaemia. You need to be able to interpret the iron study results accurately to come to this conclusion (fact sheets, p. 121). It is essential to do this prior to starting the dialogue in order to take an appropriately focussed history from this patient.

Consultation	Commentary
Doctor: Mrs. Tinker? **Mrs. Tinker:** Yes?	Checks correct patient and introduces self.
Doctor: I'm Dr. Smith. Dr. Hamad has written and asked us to see you. She has told us quite a bit about what has been happening to you and she has also sent us your recent blood test results. **Mrs. Tinker:** Oh yes.	Scene setting.
Doctor: It would be helpful if you could tell me in your own words what has been happening to you.	Open question encourages dialogue.
Mrs. Tinker: Well. I've given blood every 6 months for the last 5 years. I started doing this after my niece developed leukaemia and had to have lots of blood transfusions and a bone marrow transplant. I give blood every 6 months, but I missed	Allow patient to give account in own words.

my last donation, as I couldn't keep the appointment as I was on holiday.

So anyway, I went to give blood as usual last month, but they wouldn't let me give any. They told me I was anaemic and that I needed all my own blood and I couldn't afford to give it to anybody else.

This implies recent onset anaemia and makes coeliac disease and menorrhagia less likely causes.

They told me to go and see my own doctor. I did. She is very nice. She took some more blood tests from me and I went back to see her about 2 weeks ago for the results. She has told me I am deficient in iron. I don't understand why. I eat a very healthy diet. I eat plenty of spinach and greens and have liver and onions every Monday.

Don't interrupt until she has finished her story.

Dr. Hamad asked me a lot of questions. I have being feeling a bit tired recently. But I have a hectic life with two teenage children and a fulltime job. I'm knackered when I get home from work but I thought it was because I have been so very busy at work recently.

Patient's agenda 1.

Anyway, Dr. Hamad asked me to come to this clinic. She has told me it is a stomach and bowel clinic. I am not sure why she has sent me here, as I don't have anything wrong with my stomach or bowels. I asked her about this and she said this was the correct clinic to come to. I'm still not sure about that, but she is a good doctor and I trust her so here I am. Shouldn't I be seeing a blood specialist doctor?

Patient's agenda 2.

Doctor: Mrs. Tinker, I think Dr. Hamad was quite right to send you to this clinic. As you know your blood tests have shown you to be deficient in iron. There are a number of reasons why this might be. Some patients do not take enough iron in their diet. Some patients can't absorb enough iron

It is correct to address the patient's agenda at this point, as it informs the rest of the consultation.

from the diet. Other patients loose blood from the gut. When this happens the patient may not realise it, as often there is minor seepage of blood over a period of time. This may not produce any symptoms at all apart from the anaemia.

Mrs. Tinker: Oh, I see why I am here now.

Doctor: Some patients get breathless or swollen ankles when they become anaemic. Has this happened to you?

Closed question to determine functional consequence of the anaemia.

Mrs. Tinker: No.

Doctor: Have you noticed any other symptoms?

This patient has got asymptomatic iron deficiency anaemia.

Mrs. Tinker: Well, I just feel a bit tired. Apart from that I feel absolutely fine.

Doctor: Okay. Just let me summarise so far. You were found to be anaemic when you went to give blood but apart from a little tiredness you feel fine. *(Pause)* The blood tests that you have had show you to be deficient in iron. Does that sound right to you?

Summarise.

'Chunk and check'.

Mrs. Tinker: Yes.

Doctor: I see. I need to ask you a number of questions now to see if I can work out what may have caused your anaemia. Is that okay?

This sets the scene to ask specific questions.

Mrs. Tinker: Yes.

Doctor: Can you tell me how your periods have been over the last year or two?

Excludes a gynaecological cause for the anaemia.

Mrs. Tinker: I had a hysterectomy 10 years ago as my periods were very painful because of fibroids. I have not had a period since.

Doctor: I know it's sometime ago, but can you tell me how old you were when you started your periods?

This makes coeliac disease less likely, as such patients usually have a delayed menarche.

Mrs. Tinker: I was 11 years old.	
Doctor: I see . . . . *pause* . . . Have you had any:	No GI symptoms does not exclude significant GI pathology.
• Abdominal pain? No.	
• Loss of appetite? No.	
• Weight loss? No.	
• Swallowing difficulty? No.	
• Change in your bowel habits? No.	
• Blood in your motions? No.	
• Do you check for this regularly? No.	
Doctor: Okay. Have you noticed any blood in the urine?	Makes urological malignancy unlikely.
Mrs. Tinker: No.	
Doctor: You mentioned that you take a balanced diet, please could you tell me more about your diet?	Excludes a dietary cause.
Mrs. Tinker: Yes. I have a Mediterranean style diet with plenty of fresh fruit and vegetables. I eat meat three times a week and have fish at least two times per week. I do not eat any junk food if I can help it.	
Doctor: Have you had any:	This makes Crohn's and coeliac disease less likely.
• Mouth ulceration? No.	
• Aching in the joints? No.	
• A gritty feeling in the eyes? No.	
Doctor: Apart from your hysterectomy, have you had any other operations or illness?	This demonstrates to the patient and examiner that you have been listening.
Mrs. Tinker: No, none at all.	
Doctor: What tablets or medicines are you taking just now?	e.g. non-steroidals.
Mrs. Tinker: Dr. Hamad started me on iron tablets when I went back to see her 2 weeks ago. I've been taking three tablets per day. Since I have been taking them my motions have gone black.	Iron studies correctly taken before starting iron. Iron sends the stool black. Not to be confused with colonic blood loss.
Doctor: Are your parents both alive and well?	
Mrs. Tinker: No. My mum is 69 and as fit as a flea. My dad died at the age of 42 from bowel cancer.	This patient's lifetime risk of developing colorectal cancer is about 1 in 10.

Doctor: I'm sorry to hear that. Has anybody else in the family suffered with bowel cancer?

Mrs. Tinker: No.

Doctor: Do you:

- Smoke? No.
- Drink alcohol? No.

Doctor: What is your job?

Mrs. Tinker: I am a dinner lady at the local primary school.

Doctor: Okay. Thanks for that. Just let me summarise to check I have everything straight.

    You feel perfectly well apart from a little tiredness. You went to give blood but were refused because you were anaemic. The blood tests that you have had show you to be deficient in iron. You have recently started on iron and your stool has turned black.

    You have had no symptoms from your bowel or stomach. You have a good appetite and take a balanced diet. You had a hysterectomy 10 years ago. Your father died of colon cancer in his early 40s.

    Is that an accurate summary, or have I missed anything out?

Mrs. Tinker: Yes.

Doctor: Is there anything else that you think may be important that we haven't discussed?

Mrs. Tinker: No. I can't think of anything else

Summarise

'Chunk and check'.

This signals to the patient that the consultation is about to change from information gathering to information giving.

By now you should have a firm idea in your mind about the likely diagnosis. At the start of the consultation the differential diagnosis was quite wide. After taking the history, some of the diagnostic possibilities have become far less likely. This includes a gynaecological cause for the anaemia as the patient had a hysterectomy 10 years ago. Coeliac disease is also very unlikely as the patient has not had a chronic anaemia (regular blood donation precludes this), nor has she had any associated symptoms such as mouth ulceration, skin rashes or a delayed menarche.

The most likely cause of this patient's anaemia in view of her family history is colorectal cancer. Her father died from this condition in his 40's, and may well have had hereditary non-poylposis colorectal cancer (HNPCC). This is an autosomal dominant condition that results in colorectal cancer presenting in the 30's or early 40's. The cancers are frequently found in the right side of the colon. Remember that the most common mode of presentation of carcinoma of the caecum is an asymptomatic iron deficiency anaemia. Colonic symptoms such as obstruction imply advanced disease.

The diagnosis cannot be made on the basis of the history alone. It is now time to complete the task you have been set, and explain to the patient what the plan of investigation is going to be to elucidate the cause of her anaemia. Before you do this it is vital to tell the examiner and the patient that in normal circumstances you would perform a careful clinical examination with particular attention to the abdomen, including a rectal examination. She then needs some further blood tests including B_{12}, folate, ESR and CRP. Following this she needs an upper GI endoscopy, duodenal biopsies and a colonscopy. Ideally these endoscopic examinations should be performed at the same sitting.

Consultation	Commentary
Doctor: What has your doctor told you about what may have caused your anaemia and what tests you may need to try to find the cause?	Checks prior knowledge.
Mrs. Tinker: Nothing really. She just asked me to attend this clinic to see you.	
Doctor: As I mentioned earlier you have anaemia because of not enough iron in your system. There are quite a number of things that can cause lack of iron.	Nicely paced explanation in bite-sized pieces.
(pause)	
The commonest cause in a patient your age is because of blood loss from heavy periods, but clearly this doesn't apply to you as you had a hysterectomy 10 years ago.	

Mrs. Tinker: I see.

Doctor: Some patients don't take enough in the diet. Again, this doesn't seem to apply to you as you have a healthy balanced diet, which sounds as though it contains as much iron as your body would normally require.

Explain at pace the patient can handle.

Allow opportunity to ask questions and to clarify.

Mrs. Tinker: I see.

Doctor: Other patients don't absorb enough iron from the diet. Some patients lose iron into the bowel without realising it. If the blood oozes slowly over a period of time this can cause a patient to become anaemic. I am wondering if either of these could explain your anaemia.

Mrs. Tinker: Yes.

Doctor: To try to work this out I need to arrange for you to have some further blood tests to see if you are correctly absorbing other vitamins from the diet. I will arrange for you to have these blood tests this afternoon when we are finished if that's okay with you.

Mrs. Tinker: Yes doctor

Doctor: The other tests you need are to check if you are losing blood from the stomach or bowel without realising it.

Mrs. Tinker: Okay.

At this point, the consultation can cover the appropriate investigations required, i.e. gastrointestinal endoscopy and colonscopy. These are covered in detail as fact sheets in Chapter 8.

Time should be given to explain these tests, allowing for questions. In addition, the candidate should be prepared to discuss the possibility of cancer if the patient asks about it.

Once this is done, the consultation should be closed with a summing up and clarification of what happens next.

Consultaton	Commentary
Doctor: Okay. To summarise then. You will need some blood tests now to check you are absorbing your other vitamins. The appointments for your endoscopy will come through the post. Any queries in the meantime, give that number a ring. I'll drop a note to Dr. Hamad to let her know the plan. **Mrs. Tinker:** Thanks very much doctor.	Chunk and check

---

Fact sheet: Causes of a microcytic anaemia

This means patients who have a low haemoglobin and a low mean cell volume (MCV). Causes include:

- iron deficiency anaemia
- anaemia of chronic disorders
- β-thalassaemia trait
- sideroblastic anaemia.

The commonest cause of a microcytic anaemia is iron deficiency. There are, however, a number of other causes outlined above. It is a major mistake to assume that a microcytic anaemia is due to iron deficiency, and it is essential that in every case iron studies are performed to confirm the diagnosis prior to commencing iron therapy. Patients who have documented iron deficiency usually require invasive gastrointestinal investigations to determine the cause of their anaemia. Patients who have a microcytic anaemia due to one of the other causes usually do not require such tests.

It is also important to arrange for the iron studies to be performed **before** the patient is commenced on oral iron therapy, as such treatment will interfere with the results and make it impossible to interpret the iron studies accurately.

Fact sheet: Interpreting iron study results

Test	Iron deficiency	Anaemia of chronic disorders
Ferritin	Low*	Normal or increased
Iron saturation	Low	Normal or increased
Transferrin	High	Normal
Iron	Low	Normal or increased

*Ferritin is an 'acute phase protein', and will go up when the patient is sick from any cause. Serum ferritin can therefore sometimes be normal in patients with iron deficiency anaemia in the acute phase of an illness. The other parameters in the above table are not affected in this way and should be employed to sort out cases where there is any doubt.

Fact sheet: Clues to causes of iron deficiency anaemia

Category	Causes	Important points in history

Menstrual blood loss	Menorrhagia
	Other intra-uterine
	  pathology
		Full gynaecological
		  history is mandatory
		  in female patients

Gastrointestinal blood
  loss
	Colorectal cancer
	Stomach cancer
	Peptic ulceration
	Small bowel
		Change in bowel habit
		Rectal bleeding
		Family history
		Anorexia
		Weight loss
		Epigastric pain
		Epigastric pain related to
		  meals
		Rare

Blood loss from other
  sources
	Urological tumours,
	  e.g. cancer of the
	  bladder or kidney
		Patients usually have
		  macroscopic
		  haematuria. Sometimes
		  blood in the urine is
		  only detected after
		  dipstick testing
		  (microscopic haematuria)

Dietary	Vegetarianism Veganism Malnutrition	Full dietary history is essential

---

Fact sheet: Clues to causes of iron deficiency anaemia—cont'd

Malabsorption of iron	Coeliac disease	Recurrent mouth ulcers
		Skin rashes
		Delayed menarche
		Recurrent anaemia
	Crohn's disease	Abdominal pain
		Diarrhoea
		Mouth ulcers
		Arthralgia
	Bacterial overgrowth	Previous GI surgery
		Diarrhoea
		More common in diabetics
Unknown		After complete investigation the cause remains obscure in up to 25% of patients

Note: the commonest cause of iron deficiency anaemia in a pre-menopausal woman is excessive blood loss due to menorrhagia.

Fact sheet: Investigation of iron deficiency anaemia

- Confirm the diagnosis of iron deficiency anaemia by full blood count and iron studies (fact sheets, p. 121).
- Take a detailed history (fact sheet, p. 122).
- Perform a careful clinical examination.

If the patient is male or post-menopausal female, has no menorrhagia and takes a normal diet they need gastrointestinal investigations to exclude GI blood loss or malabsorption of iron. In patients with no GI symptoms (which is the majority) the following sequence of investigations is suggested.

Haematinics and inflammatory markers
It is important to check the serum B_{12} and red cell folate, as occasionally patients have associated deficiencies in these haematinics as well. If the patient is deficient in either, this points to a small bowel cause of the anaemia such as coeliac disease. Remember that folate is primarily absorbed from the proximal small bowel (jejunum), and B_{12} from the terminal ileum.

A raised ESR and CRP are found in gastrointestinal malignancies and small bowel Crohn's disease.

Antiendomysial antibodies
These are 99% sensitive and specific for coeliac disease. The commonest way in which coeliac disease presents in the 21st century is recurrent iron deficiency anaemia. Diarrhoea and malabsorption occur in only a minority. Patients often complain of recurrent mouth ulceration and may have suffered with recurrent skin rashes on the arm and the back (dermatitis herpetiformis) for many years. The diagnosis is confirmed by taking biopsies from the second part of the duodenum at OGD.

Fact sheet: Investigation of iron deficiency anaemia—cont'd

Upper GI endoscopy and duodenal biopsies

To exclude coeliac disease, cancer and peptic ulceration of the upper GI tract.

Colonic imaging

This is performed to exclude colorectal cancer as a cause for the iron deficiency. Remember that most patients with carcinoma of the caecum have no lower GI symptoms and usually present with asymptomatic iron deficiency anaemia. There are a number of ways of imaging the colon which include:

- colonoscopy
- flexible sigmoidoscopy and barium enema
- barium enema
- CT scan.

Elderly and infirm patients tolerate invasive procedures less well, particularly those requiring purgative bowel preparation. For this reason, elderly/infirm patients are usually investigated by CT in the first instance.

Small bowel studies

A small bowel cause for anaemia is less common. Small bowel investigations are usually reserved for patients with negative upper and lower gastrointestinal studies who have recurrent and or very severe iron deficiency anaemia. The traditional method of imaging is a small bowel barium study (either a small bowel meal and follow-through, or a small bowel enema). Unfortunately, the diagnostic pick-up rate of these studies in this situation is very poor (approximately 1%). A new method of small bowel imaging which is rapidly superseding small bowel barium X-rays is capsule endoscopy. In this test a small capsule containing a camera is swallowed. The camera takes two images per second as it passes down the small bowel. These pictures are transmitted to a recording device carried on a belt and worn by the patient. These images are downloaded onto a computer and then interrogated using special software. This results in video footage of the whole of the small bowel mucosa with an image resolution of less than 0.1 mm. This technique is user-friendly and has a diagnostic pick-up rate approaching 60%.

Role of faecal occult blood testing

Faecal occult blood testing has no role to play in the investigation of iron deficiency anaemia. They can be misleading and unhelpful as they have a significant false negative rate. In other words, an asymptomatic patient with iron deficiency anaemia needs invasive GI investigations whatever the result of the faecal occult blood tests. Faecal occult blood testing has therefore been largely abandoned. They may have a future role in screening for colorectal cancer.

14

Jaundice

You have been asked to see an 82-year-old man with jaundice. The GP's referral letter is as follows:

Dear Dr.
Thank you for seeing Mr. Jones who is an 82-year-old man who has a 2-week history of jaundice. He has never really got over the death of his wife 6 months ago. He has had mild hypertension for 10 years, which has been well controlled with bendrofluazide for the last 5 years. On examination he is obviously jaundiced and has a palpable gallbladder.
Thank you for your help.
Kind regards,

Dr. Smith
Local General Practitioner

Please take a focussed history from this patient in order to:

- Determine the most likely differential diagnosis.
- Explain the plan of investigation to the patient.

Essential skills required

- Professional, sensitive approach.
- Knowledge of differential diagnosis of jaundice in an 82-year-old.
- Awareness of exploring hidden agenda.

Think list

Your agenda
- Take a clear focussed history.
- Formulate a differential diagnosis.

Mr. Jones' agenda
- Doesn't know what is wrong with him.
- Only experience of jaundice

- Pick up on cues from Mr. Jones.
- Explain plan of action.

was a comrade in Second World War who developed infectious hepatitis in Egypt.
- Depressed following death of wife 6 months ago.
- She died of MRSA sepsis following an elective operation and he will not be treated as an in-patient whatever happens.

Danger! Common pitfalls

✗ Lack of knowledge of differential diagnosis and presentation of jaundice.
✗ Failure to pick up on Mr. Jones' agenda.
✗ Failure to address concerns and respond to cues.
✗ Failure to respect Mr. Jones' anxieties and desire to remain an outpatient.

Before you start this consultation, two communication skills 'red flags' have been waved and it is important to recognise these before you start:

- The patient has a palpable gallbladder. He may have carcinoma of the pancreas (Courvoisier's law, fact sheet, p. 134). This consultation may, therefore, involve using some of your breaking-bad-news skills.
- The patient is still grieving for his wife. You need to recognise that bereaved elderly patients are at significant risk of organic disease (as in this case), as well as depression. Furthermore, this recent major life event is likely to have had a significant influence on the patient's agenda. This may need careful handling to uncover and deal with.

This consultation is, therefore, quite complex and is certainly one of the harder communication skills tasks that you are likely to encounter in Final MB. Not only do you have to take an appropriate, focussed history relating to the jaundice, but you may need to use your breaking-bad-news skills and your skills at uncovering the patient's agenda in order to appropriately explain the plan of action.

Consultation	Commentary
Doctor: Mr. Jones? **Mr. Jones:** Yes? **Doctor:** Hello. My name is Dr. Stevens. I wonder if I could talk to you please? I have a letter from your doctor, Dr. Smith. **Mr. Jones:** Yes. **Doctor:** He's told me quite a bit about you, but could you tell me in your own words what has been happening to you?	Checks correct patient and introduces self.
Mr. Jones: I'm not sure where to begin. (*Pause*) I've not been quite right since my Gladys died last year . . . (*pause*) . . . She died in here you know . . . (*pause*) . . . She came for a new hip and caught that super bug . . . They tried all sorts of antibiotics but it was no good . . . (*pause*) . . . Her heart gave out in the end . . . (*pause*) . . . We were married 58 years . . . (*pause*) . . . I'll never get over it. I don't really want to be here doctor, as I said I would never set foot in this place again. (*Long pause*)	Do **not** interrupt the patient at this stage. Let him tell you the whole story. Encourage with eye contact, head nodding and 'mm', 'yes' and 'I see'. Patient's agenda starting to emerge. A good student would make a mental note to come back to this issue but would not interrupt at this stage.
I have managed on my own, quite well since she died. My son and his wife have been as good as gold. They only live round the corner from me but they are always there when I need them. They cook my supper every night and do my shopping every week. I do not know what I would have done if it weren't for them. (*Long pause*)	You are still nowhere near the topic of jaundice but you need to be patient.
I was okay until 3 weeks ago. My water seemed to go very dark and my motions turned a light clay colour. Mary, my daughter-in law, noticed that I had got the yellow jaundice. The jaundice seems to	At last—symptoms of progressive obstructive jaundice over 2 weeks.

have got worse. My water is very dark and I seem to have lost my interest in food.

(Long pause)

Doctor: Yes, I see. Have you had any other symptoms at all?

Mr. Jones: I may have lost a bit of weight, but not very much. I am off my food a bit, but Mary is a very good cook . . .

Doctor: How much weight have you lost?

Mr. Jones: Half a stone.

Doctor: Have you had pain in your tummy?

Mr. Jones: No.

Doctor: Have you had a fever or shaking attacks in the last 2 or 3 weeks?

Mr. Jones: No.

Doctor: Have you had jaundice before?

Mr. Jones: No. The only time I've ever seen anybody with yellow jaundice was Tommy Jarvis in Egypt in the Second World War. He was put in the isolation camp because he was infectious.

Doctor: Have you had any other illnesses or operations?

Mr. Jones: No.

Doctor: Do you take any tablets on a regular basis?

Mr. Jones: Yes. Bendrofluazide for blood pressure. I've been on them for years.

Doctor: Do you take any other medicines at all?

Mr. Jones: No.

Doctor: You have not taken any antibiotics, arthritis tablets or any herbal or non-prescription

---

You are now only two minutes into the consult. If the pause lasts you can now interject with another open question.

Open question allows you to explore patient's agenda.

Weight loss suggests malignancy.

Important closed question.

Painless jaundice makes gallstones less likely.

Absence of fever makes CBD stone unlikely.

Patient's agenda.

Patients often regard hypertension as insignificant.

Good series of questions to exclude drug-induced jaundice.

medicines at all in the last 2 months? **Mr. Jones:** No. **Doctor:** Are you allergic to any tablets or medicines? **Mr. Jones:** No. **Doctor:** Have you ever smoked? **Mr. Jones:** No. **Doctor:** How much alcohol do you drink in an average week? **Mr. Jones:** I go to the Crown on Wednesday's for quiz night and have two pints of beer. I go to the British Legion on Saturdays and have two pints of beer then as well. **Doctor:** Have you ever drunk more than this? **Mr. Jones:** No. I've never been a big drinker. **Doctor:** I guess you've been retired for some time. What was your job? **Mr. Jones:** I was a plumber all my life.	Excludes possibility of alcoholic hepatitis.

You are now about 5 minutes into the consultation. You should know by now that the likely diagnosis is carcinoma of the head of the pancreas, as the patient has had a brief history of painless jaundice, has lost weight and has a palpable gallbladder. It is unlikely that he has had a common bile duct stone, as he has had no pain or fever. He could have metastatic liver disease, but the gallbladder should not be palpable, but it is possible that the GP has made an error, as this is not a common clinical sign. It is unlikely that the patient has alcohol or drug-related hepatitis on the basis of the history you have taken.

To complete the history you would need to ask about the following:

- recent travel
- blood transfusions
- tattoos
- infectious contacts
- sexual history
- recreational drugs, etc.

These are largely to exclude acute and chronic viral liver disease.

In the context of this particular patient these subjects are less relevant, as viral hepatitis is uncommon at this age. A good student would now go back to the two 'red flag' communication issues, which are:

- Patient's agenda surrounding the death of his wife.
- Explain the plan of investigation to the patient in the light of the above and taking into account that the patient may possibly have a carcinoma of the head of the pancreas.

The correct question to ask now is therefore something like:

Doctor: I know that this may be painful for you but would you be able to tell me more about what happened to your wife?

This results in uncovering the patient's agenda that he will, under no circumstances, be admitted overnight to hospital. He does agree, however, to be investigated on an outpatient basis.

You now need to complete your task, which is to explain the likely diagnosis and plan of investigations.

Consultation	Commentary
Doctor: What has your doctor told you about what may have caused your jaundice?	Check prior knowledge.
Mr. Jones: Not much. He insisted I came here to see you. I did not want to after what happened to my wife. No offence meant doctor! I told him I would not allow myself to be admitted.	
Doctor: Yes. I understand that. Have you any idea what may have caused the jaundice?	Check prior knowledge again and explore any concerns.
Mr. Jones: I wondered whether I had the same as Tommy Jarvis all those years ago.	

Doctor: It is possible, but from what you have told me I think it is very unlikely.

(Pause)

Mr. Jones: Why's that doctor?

Doctor: What Tommy had all those years ago was almost certainly a viral infection of the liver called hepatitis A. That particular infection is extremely rare in a patient your age.

Mr. Jones: Does that mean I'm not infectious?

Another part of patient's agenda emerging.

Doctor: I think that is extremely unlikely, as I do not think an infection of your liver is the cause of your jaundice

Mr. Jones: What do you think is the matter with me then doctor?

Doctor: I'm not completely sure.

Mr. Jones: You must have some idea doctor!

Doctor: It is possible that you have a blockage to the bile duct as it drains from the liver

Extra marks for a diagram of biliary tree.

Mr. Jones: Oh, I see.

Doctor: The first thing to do is to confirm that the pipe is blocked, and if it is we need to unblock it. You should understand that being an ex-plumber.

Relating to patient's prior knowledge.

Mr. Jones: How will you do that?

Doctor: You will need a special blood test, which I will arrange to have taken in a few moments. *(Pause)* As you do not want to come into hospital I will arrange for you to have a test called an ultrasound scan as an outpatient, maybe tomorrow. *(Pause)* These two tests will tell us whether the bile duct is blocked.

Frequent pauses to allow for questions, clarification and pick up on non-verbal cues.

Mr. Jones: What will happen if it is? How can you unblock it?

Doctor: There are a number of ways in which this can be done, and it may be possible to do this as an outpatient if necessary. I will need to get you an appointment to discuss things with a specialist first though.

Mr. Jones: I see.

Doctor: I know this is quite a bit to take in all at once. Have you any questions you would like to ask me at this stage?

Demonstrates empathy. Offer chance to clarify.

Mr. Jones: I don't think so doctor thank you.

Doctor: Just to summarise, then. *(Pause)* I think you may have a blockage of the bile duct, which has caused your jaundice. *(Pause)* I am not sure what has caused this. *(Pause)* You need to have a blood test now and an ultrasound scan tomorrow to confirm that the bile duct is blocked . . . *(pause)* . . . and what may have caused it. *(Pause)* . . . You are not infectious and you do not need to stay in hospital if you don't want to. *(Pause)* I will arrange for you to see a specialist later this week to discuss the results of the scan and blood tests. *(Pause)* With your permission I will tell him that you do not want to be admitted to hospital overnight if the bile duct needs unblocking.

Once again, allow frequent pauses to give opportunity for questions, clarification and to pick up non-verbal cues.

Mr. Jones: Okay doctor.

Doctor: Is there anything else you would like to ask?

Bringing consultation to close.

Mr. Jones: No. I don't think so.

Doctor: Well, we'll get these tests done and then arrange to see you with the results.

It is generally safe to manage patients with obstructive jaundice in the community providing they do not have any evidence of cholangitis, so long as they are investigated and treated very promptly. Patients with cholangitis should be admitted to hospital for intravenous fluids and antibiotics.

Common causes of jaundice in an 82-year-old man

Cause	Symptoms	Signs
Carcinoma of the pancreas	Painless (usually) Weight loss	Jaundice May have palpable gallbladder[Courvoisier's law, p.134]
Common bile duct stone	Painful	Jaundice Abdominal tenderness Fever[Charcot's triad, p. 134]
Metastatic liver disease	May have pain from inflammation of liver capsule Very significant weight loss	Jaundice Rock hard craggy liver edge
Alcoholic hepatitis	Significant alcohol history	Signs of chronic liver disease
Drug-induced jaundice	History of recent new drug therapy especially: • antibiotics • NSAIDs	Jaundice May have hepatomegaly

Uncommon causes of jaundice in an 82-year-old man

Cause	Symptoms	Notes
Decompensated chronic liver disease • alcoholic • chronic viral hepatitis (B&C) • PSC • haemochromatosis • autoimmune	Abdominal swelling due to ascites Encephalopathy Sepsis	Always ask **why** the patient has decompensated • sepsis • spontaneous bacterial peritonitis • GI bleed • constipation • hepatoma
Acute viral hepatitis	Flu-like illness Incubation 2–6 weeks Need travel (A,B&E), sexual (B&C), and dietary (A&E) history	Acute viral hepatitis is rare in patients over the age of 50 years Need to take accurate immunisation history
Recreational drugs	Easily missed if not enquired about	Very rare at this age Ecstasy induced liver damage is common in young
Right heart failure	Patients are always breathless	Jaundice is mild and patient has a pulsatile liver and a very raised JVP
Haemolysis	Tired pale and jaundiced	Will be anaemic Uncommon in this age group

Fact sheet: Courvoisier's law

This was first described by the French physician Courvoisier over 100 years ago, and is still relevant in the 21st century. Courvoisier's law states that:

'In the presence of jaundice a palpable gallbladder is not due to stones.'

The two common causes of obstructive jaundice are:

- pancreatico-biliary carcinoma (usually carcinoma of the head of pancreas)
- common bile duct stones.

In both conditions, because of the biliary obstruction, the pressure in the biliary system goes up as the bile cannot escape via the bile duct into the second part of the duodenum. When this is caused by a stone impacted in the distal common bile duct, the gallbladder does not enlarge. The reason for this is that, although the pressure in the gallbladder may go up, the gallbladder cannot expand and become palpable. This is because in patients with gallstone disease the gallbladder is chronically inflamed and fibrosed. The gallbladder in this situation is therefore non-compliant and will not enlarge even if the pressure within is significantly raised.

In contrast, patients with a malignant distal common duct stricture have a thin-walled compliant gallbladder. When the pressure in the biliary system goes up due to the blocked distal bile duct, the gallbladder can expand and sometimes becomes palpable.

Therefore, in a patient who is jaundiced and has a palpable gallbladder, the likely cause is a carcinoma of the head of the pancreas and not a common bile duct stone. The question states that the patient has a palpable gallbladder, and an understanding of Courvoisier's law should indicate that this consultation may include breaking-bad-news skills and is not just about taking a structured jaundice history.

Fact sheet: Charcot's triad

Charcot invented his triad in the 19th century. It is still of great value in modern medicine. Charcot's triad is a combination of three symptoms:

- jaundice
- abdominal pain
- fever.

When these symptoms occur together this indicates that the patient has got cholangitis, i.e. has an infection in the bile duct. In a patient with no prior biliary history this is nearly always due to a stone in the common bile duct.

15

Chest pain

Roger Weeks, a 45-year-old man with chest pain, is referred to you by the Accident and Emergency Department. The doctor who saw the patient says his ECG looks normal.

Please take a structured history from this patient and formulate:

- a differential diagnosis
- a management plan.

Essential skills required

- Knowledge of differential diagnosis of chest pain in a 45-year-old man (fact sheet, p. 140).
- Knowledge of the appropriate management of patients with chest pain (fact sheet, p. 143).
- Generic consultation skills.

Think list

Doctor's agenda
- Take an accurate pain history (fact sheet, p. 143).
- Knowledge of differential diagnosis of chest pain.
- Knowledge of management of chest pain.

Mr. Weeks' agenda
- Patient is not sure what all the fuss is about. He is now pain free.
- He wants to leave in 45 minutes as he is the captain of the village cricket team which is playing in the county village cup final this afternoon at 2 pm.

Danger! Common pitfalls

✗ Lack of knowledge.
✗ Misuse of leading questions.
✗ Not addressing Mr. Weeks' agenda, i.e. his cricket match.

Misuse of leading questions

In order to ascertain the cause of chest pain, you will need to illicit specific details from the patient. There is a danger of asking leading questions:

Doctor:	Is the pain a crushing sensation that radiates down your left arm?
Mr. Weeks:	Um . . . yes.

Likewise, the way we ask the question may influence the answer; so avoid directing the patient to a particular response.

Doctor:	You don't get any palpitations do you?
Mr. Weeks:	Um . . . no.

For the sake of the exam, it is best to start with an open-ended question and then follow it with something more specific. This way you demonstrate to the examiner the use of open questions but then can direct the patient to specific details.

Doctor:	Does the pain go anywhere else?
Mr. Weeks:	I'm not sure.
Doctor:	Does the pain go down your arm?
Mr. Weeks:	Oh, yes. It's more like pins and needles.

This way you demonstrate to the examiner the use of open questions but then can direct the patient to specific details.

Example answer

Consultation	Commentary
Doctor: Mr. Roger Weeks? **Mr. Weeks:** Yes.	Checks identity.
Doctor: Hello, I'm Dr. Adams. **Mr. Weeks:** Hello.	Introduces self.

Doctor: I've been asked to come and talk to you about this chest pain you have had. Could you tell me in your own words what has been happening to you?

Open question.

Mr. Weeks: Okay. I'm not sure what all the fuss is about really. I was doing some gardening this morning and I got a bit of pain in the middle of my chest. Just a niggle really. I think I may have pulled a muscle when I was digging. Anyway, I stopped gardening and sat down for about half-an-hour. The pain went off.

Patients agenda 1.

Listening skills.

Allow patient to give a account.

Judy, my wife, panicked a bit I think. She works as a doctor's receptionist. She called 999 and an ambulance came to pick me up and here I am. The pain has gone. I think I strained a muscle. The other doctor says my ECG was normal, so can I go now please, doctor, as I have a very important cricket match at 2 o'clock.

Clear indication from patient that he doesn't wish to stay.

Doctor: I just need to clarify a few things first, just to check that it is only a muscle strain and not anything more serious. Would that be okay?

Mr. Weeks: Of course, doctor.

Communicates that patient's agenda has been heard.

Doctor: Patients often find describing the quality of pain quite difficult. Could you please describe in your own words exactly what the pain you had felt like?

Clarifying open question.

Mr. Weeks: It was in the middle of my chest. It felt dull. It lasted about half-an-hour. It was as though someone was sitting on my chest.

Very suggestive of cardiac pain.

Doctor: I see . . . *(pause)*. . .

Mr. Weeks: That's about it really. I sat down on the wall and after 30 minutes the pain went on its own.

Doctor: Is there anything else you can tell me about the pain?	Checking that the patient's account is complete.
Mr. Weeks: No, doctor.	
Doctor: Okay. I need to ask you a few questions about the pain so I can get it straight in my mind what we are dealing with here. Is that okay?	Signals forthcoming closed **PASQDAPE** questions.
Mr. Weeks: Yes, doctor.	
Doctor: It sounds as though the pain was in the centre of your chest.	**P**osition/radiation.
Mr. Weeks: Yes.	
Doctor: Did the pain move anywhere?	Radiation asked as open-ended question.
Mr. Weeks: No, it stayed in the middle of my chest.	
Doctor: Did it move up to your jaw or down either of your arms?	Specific enquiry to check if radiation of cardiac nature.
Mr. Weeks: No.	
Doctor: You were doing some gardening at the time?	**A**ctivity at time.
Mr. Weeks: Yes. I was digging over the potato bed.	
Doctor: Did it come on suddenly or gradually?	**S**peed of onset.
Mr. Weeks: Suddenly. I thought I pulled a muscle digging.	
Doctor: So to recap, the pain lasted 30 minutes and was dull, as though someone was sitting on your chest?	Clarification of history. **Q**uality. **D**uration.
Mr. Weeks: Yes.	
Doctor: When you got the pain did you have any other symptoms at the same time?	**A**ssociated symptoms.
Mr. Weeks: No.	
Doctor: Any breathlessness *(pause)* palpitations *(pause)*, giddiness *(pause)*, fainting *(pause)* sweating *(pause)*, nausea *(pause)* or sickness?	Pause for answer to each question.
Mr. Weeks: No, doctor.	
Doctor: Have you had a pain like this before?	**P**revious episodes.

Mr. Weeks: No, doctor.

Doctor: The pain seems as though it went after 30 minutes rest. Did you try anything else to make it go away?

Exacerbating/relieving factors.

Mr. Weeks: No, doctor.

Doctor: Did anything seem to aggravate the pain when you had it?

Mr. Weeks: How do you mean doctor?

Doctor: For example, did movement make it worse?

Mr. Weeks: No

Doctor: Was the chest tender to touch?

Mr. Weeks: No, doctor.

Doctor: I see. So let me see if I have got this right. You were digging the garden and you suddenly developed a dull central chest pain. The pain didn't move anywhere, and was dull in nature. There were no associated symptoms at the time. You have never had any similar pains. The pain got better after 30 minutes rest. Is that a reasonable summary of what has happened?

Summarise. 'Chunk and check'.

Mr. Weeks: Yes, doctor.

Doctor: Is there anything I've missed out or anything else you think may be important?

Check for any other issues. Demonstrates interest in patient's views.

Mr. Weeks: No, doctor. Do you think I have pulled a muscle in my chest doctor?

Doctor: I don't think the pain is due to muscle strain. *(pause)* From what you are telling me, I think it could be something else. I need to ask a few more questions and then we need to talk about that. Is that okay?

Answer patients question. Important not to ignore his agenda.

You now need to ask about his risk factors for developing ischaemic heart disease (fact sheet, p. 144).

It is obvious from this history that this patient's pain could be cardiac rather than musculoskeletal. This being the case he needs to be admitted to hospital for the following:

- bed rest
- serial ECGs
- serum troponin-T, 12 hours after the onset of the pain
- oral aspirin
- oral clopidogrel
- oral β-blocker
- subcutaneous low molecular weight heparin.

The rationale for adopting this approach will need to be carefully explained to the patient and in particular that his normal ECG does not necessarily exclude significant ischaemic heart disease. If the patient is still resistant to immediate in-patient care he needs to be told firmly that the symptoms that he has had could herald the onset of a full-blown and potentially fatal myocardial infarction. Playing cricket would, therefore, not be in his health's best interests.

If the patient insists on leaving, the risks must be carefully explained to the patient and documented in the patient's case notes. It is wise to ask the patient to sign a 'discharge against medical advice' form.

If the consultation focuses on the patient's insistence that he leaves, do not get confrontational with him. Don't forget that this may be his way of dealing with his own fears about his health. Denial can be a very effective coping mechanism.

Maintain your cool. Remain calm and sympathetic. Listen to his issues but clearly explain your opinion. If possible, offer to speak with his wife about the importance of staying in hospital.

Fact sheet: Differential diagnosis of chest pain	
Causes	*Symptoms*
Cardiac • Angina	• Acute onset, dull, central, crushing • Effort-related, but not always • Radiates to jaw and down the arms • Associated with sweating, nausea • Duration: variable (minutes to 1 hour)

Fact sheet: Differential diagnosis of chest pain—cont'd

Causes	Symptoms
Cardiac—cont'd • Myocardial infarction	• Acute onset, dull, central, crushing • Not necessarily related to effort • Radiates to jaw and down the arms • Associated with sweating, breathlessness and vomiting • Duration: hours, until analgesia given
Pleuritic • Pneumothorax • Pulmonary embolus • Viral pleurisy • Pneumonia	• Acute onset: PE and pneumothorax • Onset over days: viral and pneumonic pleurisy • Unilateral pain; sharp and stabbing • No radiation • Worse with coughing and deep inspiration • Associated with breathlessness, particularly PE
Musculoskeletal	• Acute onset; unilateral, sometimes central • Worse with movement, especially twisting • No associated symptoms • Patient may remember physical trigger • Patient may complain of chest wall tenderness
Oesophageal • Reflux disease • Oesophageal spasm	• Patients usually have chronic symptoms, and this may be an acute flare of a long-standing problem • Central, burning; radiates up to jaw or into back • Worse when lying flat or stooping • Often precipitated by a late heavy meal • May have associated water brash (acid taste in the mouth) • Acute, central; dull or sharp • Radiates to back, sometime the jaw • Duration minutes to hours • May have associated reflux disease • Can be difficult to distinguish from cardiac disease, and is often relieved by GTN • Commonly starts in patients in their 40's
Idiopathic • 'Non-specific chest pain'	• Common • May have some of the features of all of the above

Fact sheet: Differential diagnosis of chest pain—cont'd	
Causes	*Symptoms*
	• Diagnosis by exclusion, but an experienced physician can 'smell' these cases • Prognosis is good as there is no demonstrable pathology
Note: the speed of onset of symptoms is often not given the importance it deserves in medical texts. For example, sudden onset of acute pleuritic pain and breathlessness with a normal chest X-ray is a pulmonary embolism until proven otherwise	

Fact sheet: Uncommon causes of chest pain	
Causes	*Symptoms*
Pericardial • Viral pericarditis	• Sub-acute onset (hours–days) • Sharp, central; positionally dependent • Worse on deep inspiration/expiration • No radiation • May have had preceding flu-like symptoms; no other associated symptoms
Aortic • Acute dissection of the thoracic aorta	• Very uncommon; an important diagnosis to make • Often mistaken for an acute MI with disastrous consequences (thrombolytic therapy will kill a patient with a dissection) • Hyper-acute onset of severe pain • Central, radiating through to the back • Dull and ripping in nature • Patient cannot find a comfortable position and wriggles in the bed • Usually have a history of hypertension • Duration: hours
Abdominal • Acute pancreatitis • Perforated DU • Peptic ulcer • Biliary colic • Abdominal aortic aneurysm	• Can present as lower chest pain • Careful clinical assessment and understanding that pathology below the diaphragm can occasionally produce chest pain is required to achieve an accurate diagnosis

Fact sheet: Clinical management of chest pain

This is a very common clinical problem, and is likely to be one you will encounter from day one of your career as a doctor.

Step 1: Take an accurate and focussed history (fact sheet, below).

Step 2: Perform a detailed clinical examination with particular attention to cardiovascular and respiratory system. There are often limited or no clinical signs.

Step 3: Special investigations. These may include:
- ECGs
- CXR
- blood gases
- FBC
- cardiac enzymes
- CT chest
- CT pulmonary angiogram
- VQ scan
- exercise ECG
- coronary angiography.

The exact choice and sequence of investigations depends on the clinical situation and the resources available locally.

Step 4: Immediate therapy. In a patient with undiagnosed central chest pain, after the above steps, it is important to assume that it is cardiac until proven otherwise. Patients with ischaemic heart disease commonly experience anginal symptoms in the days prior to a myocardial infarction and it is important to be aware of this as it affects immediate management. Important aspects of management of a patient with angina include:
- bed rest
- oral aspirin
- oral clopidogrel
- oral β-blocker
- high-dose low molecular weight heparin.

If the patient continues to get ischaemic pain despite the above measures an intravenous nitrate infusion is often used.

Fact sheet: Taking an accurate and complete pain history

Patients often have difficulty in describing pain. Actually they don't. What they find difficult is describing pain in the terms in which the doctor wants to hear it! To facilitate the patient to give a full and complete account of the pain, we recommend that the following approach is adopted. It is best, as in all history taking, to start with an open question. In the setting of a patient who is trying to describe pain we would recommend the following question:

'I understand you have had some pain in your chest. Could you tell me in your own words what has been happening?'

Fact sheet: Taking an accurate and complete pain history—cont'd

Now allow the patient to tell the story in his or her own words. Do **not** interrupt, and encourage the patient with non-verbal clues such as head nodding and good eye contact. If you say anything during the patient's monologue it must be restricted to encouraging monosyllables such as 'yes' or 'mmm' or 'I see'. The aspect of the history that patients find most difficult is describing the quality of the pain. If your patient is experiencing this problem you can encourage by saying:

> 'Patients often find describing pain quite difficult. Can you liken the pain to anything that you have experienced before? For example, does the pain have a 'labour pain' quality which comes and goes a bit?'

This is a patient-friendly way of asking if the pain is colicky in nature. Once the patient has described the pain as best able, use the PASQDAPE system of closed questions to clarify/confirm and fill in the gaps.

Checklist for a pain history: **PASQDAPE**
- **P**osition and radiation
- **A**ctivity at time or just before
- **S**peed of onset
- **Q**uality
- **D**uration
- **A**ssociated symptoms
- **P**revious episodes of similar pain
- **E**xacerbating/relieving factors.

It is fairly common to see in a patient's notes the entry 'poor historian'. When this occurs it is, more often than not, a reflection of the doctor's rather than the patient's limited ability. Applying the above principles will allow you to you use the term 'poor historian' in an appropriately frugal fashion.

Fact sheet: Risk factors for ischaemic heart disease

- Smoking—past or present
- Hypertension
- Family history of ischaemic heart disease
- Hyperlipidaemia
- Obesity

16

Headache

Dear Dr.
I would be grateful for your opinion on Mr. James Farmer, a 28-year-old stockbroker who gives a 12-month history of recurrent severe headaches. Examination is completely normal.
Yours Sincerely

Dr. Partridge

Take a focussed history from Mr. Farmer. You do not need to examine him.

Essential skills required

- Knowledge of causes of headaches and ability to differentiate between them.
- Ability to obtain relevant information.
- Empathic approach.
- Anticipate and manage Mr. Farmer's concerns and questions.

Think list

Your agenda	Mr. Farmer's agenda
• Obtain clear focussed history.	• May be worried he has a brain tumour.
• Diagnose or rule out life-threatening diagnosis.	• May think referral to a specialist suggests something really *is* wrong.
• Address any questions or anxieties.	• Headaches may be affecting his work.

Danger! Common pitfalls

There are several common mistakes which students make that can be easily avoided.

✗ Lack of basic knowledge.
✗ Not checking current understanding.

✗ Use of medical jargon.

✗ Not acknowledging patient's concerns.

Before you start this consultation it is important to have a differential diagnosis as to the causes of long-term headache. These are given in the fact sheet on page 147. The majority of people who are referred with long-term headaches are terrified that they have a brain tumour. A year's history makes this diagnosis unlikely especially in the absence of focal neurological signs.

In addition to asking the relevant questions given in the fact sheet on page 148, you must ascertain Mr. Farmer's concerns. This is often easier to address once you have all the information available, having taken the focussed history.

Doctor:	Is there anything in particular you're concerned the headaches may be due to?
Mr. Farmer:	Well, I'm rather worried that I've got a brain tumour.
Doctor:	I don't think this is due to a brain tumour.
Mr. Farmer:	No?
Doctor:	Your examination is normal and the story makes a brain tumour very unlikely. *(pause)* Your headaches have been going on for 12 months now and if this were due to a tumour you would be very unwell indeed. *(pause)* Also your examination would not be normal.

It is important that as well as eliciting concerns, you address them. The patient needs to understand why you do not think he has a tumour or else he will leave the consultation dissatisfied. There is danger that you will come across as dismissive and unconcerned.

Doctor:	Is there anything in particular you're concerned the headaches may be due to?
Mr. Farmer:	Well, I'm rather worried that I've got a brain tumour.
Doctor:	I don't think this is due to a brain tumour.
Mr. Farmer:	How do you know?
Doctor:	Just trust me you don't have a tumour.
Mr. Farmer:	But . . .
Doctor:	Look, its migraine. Don't worry about it.

You will need to be flexible and tailor the consultation according to the patient. In Mr. Farmer's case it is important to ask about lifestyle, since life as a stockbroker is likely to be stressful. Ensure you ask about

- alcohol intake
- time spent on the computer
- stress
- impact of headaches on lifestyle.

The fact sheets on the following pages outline the differential diagnosis of chronic headache and essential information that should be obtained. For completeness we have also included a differential diagnosis of acute-presenting headache, should you get an emergency admission scenario.

Fact sheet: Causes of chronic headache	
Differential diagnosis	*Suggestive features*

Tumour	• Sub-acute onset with steady progression over days or weeks
	• Systemic features such as fever
	• Change in pattern or character of established headache
	• Focal neurological signs
	  — papilloedema
	  — personality change
	  — seizures

Migraine	• Unilateral or bilateral in temporal area • Constant or throbbing • Episodic with complete resolution between attacks • Take to bed with curtains closed • Nausea (90%), vomiting (75%) • Aura • Identifiable precipitants, i.e. foods, menstrual cycle
Tension-type headache	• Band-like bifronto-temporal pressure • Mild nausea and photophobia • Worsened by stress • May occur daily • May be relieved with alcohol
Cranial arteritis	• Diffuse unilateral or bilateral headache • Scalp tenderness

Fact sheet: Causes of chronic headache—cont'd	
Differential diagnosis	*Suggestive features*
	• Jaw claudication • Joint pains • Sudden onset visual disturbance • Uncommon if patient under 60 years old
Cluster headache	• Six times more common in males • Severe unilateral orbital or supra-orbital pain • Intense constant boring pain • Attack lasts up to 3 hours, occurring up to three times a day for a month • Attacks occur at the same time each day • Cluster of attacks may occur a couple of times a year • Alcohol may trigger attacks • During attack the following may be observed: — lacrimation — conjunctival injection — nasal congestion — eyelid oedema

Fact sheet: Essential questions in assessment of chronic headache	
Essential questions	*Clinical relevance*
How long have you had these headaches?	• Unlikely to be a brain tumour if headaches present for more than a year
How often do they occur and how long do they last?	• *Single discrete headache*: migraine and cluster headache • *Exacerbations with a constant background*: chronic tension headache
Where do you get the pain?	• Bilateral, frontal temporal, occipital
Describe what the pain feels like.	• *Throbbing*: migraine • *Boring, intense unilateral*: cluster headache • *Band like tightness*: tension type headache
Dose anything seem to bring the headaches on or relieve them?	• Migraine precipitated by alcohol, certain foods and menstruation • Cluster headaches relieved by alcohol during acute attack

Fact sheet: Essential questions in assessment of chronic headache—cont'd

Essential questions	Clinical relevance
Do you notice anything else when you have this headache?	• Visual phenomena with migraine • Jaw claudication with temporal arteritis • Bloodshot eye and runny nose with cluster headache
What medicines are you taking?	• Do analgesics help with the pain? • Sometimes chronic analgesic use will make chronic headaches worse
Have you had any other illnesses in the past?	• Anxiety, depression and neck trauma are relevant to tension type headache • Previous head injury, meningitis and sub-arachnoid haemorrhage may predispose to communicating hydrocephalus

Fact sheet: Causes of acute-onset severe headache

Cause	Symptoms	Signs
Meningitis	• Gradual-onset headache • Flu-like symptoms • Fever • Nausea • Sensitive to light	• Neck stiffness • Kernig's sign • Photophobia • Reduced conscious level
Sub-arachnoid haemorrhage	• Sudden-onset severe headache • Occurred during exertion • Transient loss of consciousness • Vomiting • 'Warning headache' a few days prior to presentation	• Reduced conscious level • Focal neurological signs • Neck stiffness • Hypertensive
Intra-cerebral bleed	• Sudden onset headache • Loss of consciousness • Sudden onset disability	• Reduced conscious level • Focal neurology

Note: This list is not exhaustive especially as many of the causes of chronic headache in the fact sheet on page 147 can present acutely. In particular, migraine can present acutely like a sub-arachnoid haemorrhage and should be included in the differential.

Pruritus

Mr. Sampson is a 28-year-old telephonist who rarely attends surgery. He attends with a 3-month history of itching. Take a focussed history.

Essential skills required

- Knowledge of causes of pruritus and ability to differentiate between them.
- Ability to obtain relevant information.
- Focussed approach.
- Identify and deal with potentially serious causes of pruritus.

Think list

Your agenda	Mr. Sampson's agenda
• Obtain clear focussed history.	• Itching is a nuisance.
• Diagnose or rule out serious diagnosis.	• Unlikely to think this is the sign of serious disease.
• Address any questions or anxieties.	• Sleep disturbed by itching.

Danger! Common pitfalls

There are several common mistakes which students make that can be easily avoided.

✗ Lack of basic knowledge.
✗ Unsystematic approach.
✗ Use of medical jargon.
✗ Not anticipating concerns.

Since common things are common, there is most likely to be a benign cause of his itching. However, it is vital that you consider the serious causes since it takes a lot for a patient like this to present with itch. Make sure you check for systemic symptoms including weight loss, lethargy, dyspnoea and sweats.

Fact sheet: Essential questions in assessment of pruritus	
Essential questions	*Clinical relevance*
How long have you been itching?	May coincide with other events such as starting new medicines or foreign travel
Is the itching generalised or only in specific areas?	Generalised itching suggests a systemic cause whilst localised itching is most likely due to external causes
Is the itching associated with a rash?	Presence of a rash will narrow down possible diagnoses. (See fact sheet below)
Is the itching worse at any particular time?	Itching is often worse at night but especially with scabies
Have you had any illnesses in the past?	Important to note history of anaemia, renal or hepatic disease
What medicines are you taking?	See fact sheet, p. 152 for drugs that cause pruritus
How have you been feeling recently?	General systems review is essential. Especially ask questions that will relate to features of anaemia, thyroid problems, malignancy, and renal or liver impairment
Is anyone else in the family affected?	Suggests a transmissible cause such as scabies or family history of atopy
Have you been abroad recently?	Important to consider tropical infections
How's your appetite?	This can lead into other questions to explore mood; pruritus can reflect psychiatric illness especially depression

Fact sheet: Systemic causes of pruritus
Mnemonic: **BLINKED** • **B**lood disease, e.g. iron deficiency anaemia • **L**iver disease • **I**nfection, **I**mmunological or auto**I**mmune • **N**eoplasm, e.g. lymphoma • **K**idney disease • **E**ndocrine disease, e.g. hypo/hyperthyroidism • **D**rugs (see fact sheet, p. 152)

Fact sheet: Causes of pruritus according to presence of rash

Pruritus with rash	Pruritus without rash
• Urticaria	• Obstructive liver disease
• Scabies	• Chronic renal failure
• Lichen planus	• Iron deficiency anaemia
• Dermatitis herpetiformis	• Malignancy, e.g. lymphoma
• Eczma	• Drugs (see fact sheet below)
• Bullous pemphigoid	• Polycythemia rubra vera
• Drug eruptions	• Hyper/hypothyroidism
• Insect bites	• Psychiatric

Fact sheet: Drugs causing pruritus

• Opioids
• Aspirin
• Nicatinamide
• Chloroquine
• Quinidine
• Barbiturates
• Drugs causing cholestasis: penicillin, oral contraceptive pill, chlorpromazine, imipramine

Syncope

Mr. Toby Talbot, a 76-year-old retired pest-control officer, is admitted as an emergency following a blackout. Please take a history from him and construct a differential diagnosis.

Essential skills required

- Knowledge of differential diagnosis of syncope in a 76-year-old man.
- Generic consultation skills.
- Taking a history from an eyewitness.

Think list

Your agenda	Mr. Talbot's agenda
• Obtain clear focussed history from patient and eyewitness. • Formulate differential diagnosis. • Address any questions or anxieties.	• Mr. Talbot had a brief blackout whilst shopping. He now feels fine. He is not sure what all the fuss is about. • He wants to go home and have any tests performed as an out-patient.

Danger! Common pitfalls

There are several common mistakes which students make that can be easily avoided.

- ✘ Lack of basic knowledge.
- ✘ Not checking current understanding and concerns.
- ✘ Not seeking collateral history from someone who observed the event.
- ✘ Not acknowledging his concerns/ignoring his agenda.

Syncope is defined as a loss of consciousness due to a reduction of blood flow to the brain. It is usually transitory. A blackout is defined as temporary loss of consciousness of any cause. There are a large number of causes, some of which may be life threatening and some of which are more trivial (see fact sheet below). An accurate history from the patient, regarding symptoms before and after the attack, will help you decide the likely cause and construct a differential diagnosis. However, in patients with a blackout it is vital to get as much collateral history as possible from someone who witnessed the episode. For example, the patient may have had epileptiform movements of the limbs during the attack. He will not be able to tell you this, as he will not remember the episode. An eyewitness will.

It is important to distinguish syncope or blackouts from a mechanical fall. Both are common in the elderly. These two can be readily distinguished by taking a careful history from the patient and any eyewitness. The key point is that in syncope or blackout, the patient looses consciousness and then falls to the floor.

Fact sheet: Causes of syncope	
Cause	*Symptoms*
Vasovagal • Simple faint • Prolonged standing • Cough syncope • Micturition syncope	• Simple faints may be triggered by certain environmental stimuli • Syncope preceded by light-headedness, nausea, sweating • Patient may be limp and pale during and immediately after attack • Attack aborted by lying flat

Cardiac arrhythmia
• Bradycardia
• Sinus node dysfunction
• 3rd degree a-v block
• Tachycardia
   — Ventricular
   — Supraventricular
	• May be precipitated by exercise
	• Patient may have preceding palpitations
	• May have no warning symptoms ('drop attack')
	• Patient appears pale and may be temporarily pulseless
	• As the patient recovers they may flush

Cardiac outflow obstruction • Aortic stenosis	• Syncope after exercise, e.g. climbing a flight of stairs • This is an uncommon but important cause of syncope in the elderly
Pulmonary embolus	• In the elderly a pulmonary embolus may present as syncope with no pain or dyspnoea

Fact sheet: Causes of syncope—cont'd	
Cause	*Symptoms*
	• The diagnosis is frequently overlooked • Check for risk factors for thromboembolic disease and blood gases (the patient will be hypoxic)
Vertebro-basilar • Insufficiency • Transient ischaemic attack (TIA)	• Vertebro-basilar insufficiency is caused by an interruption of the blood flow in the vertebro-basilar territory • Often precipitated by head movement • May have associated brainstem symptoms such as vertigo • Symptoms may be reproduced by carotid sinus massage • Vertebro-basilar TIAs cause similar symptoms
Postural hypotension Idiopathic Drug-induced	• Idiopathic postural hypotension is common in the elderly • Syncope on standing • Aggravated or precipitated by antihypertensive drugs and diuretics
Epilepsy	• Aura or warning symptoms • Tongue-biting • Incontinence • Tonic/clonic movements (witnessed) • Post-ictal confusion
Hypoglycaemia	• Very rare in non-diabetics
Unknown	• A substantial minority of patients have no cause found even after scrupulous investigation

As you can see from this list, there are some potentially life-threatening conditions that may be the cause of Mr. Talbot's symptoms. Allowing him home to have out-patient investigations may fulfil his immediate agenda. However, this may not ultimately be in his best interests if he suddenly drops down dead from a malignant cardiac arrhythmia before he has been properly investigated. Remember his resting ECG may be quite normal and arrhythmias may only be picked-up by prolonged ECG monitoring.

Fact sheet: Essential questions about syncope	
Essential questions	*Clinical relevance*
Can you tell me the events leading up to this funny turn?	This is the most important question and should be as open as possible. Get a full account before focussing on specific closed questions. In particular, check whether the syncope was associated with standing up, turning head or sitting down. Were these associated with micturition, cough, defecation or swallowing?
How long have these been going on for? Are they becoming more frequent?	These questions give an idea of the time frame of the problem. Many cardiac and vascular causes may have come on recently and become progressively worse
Did you have any palpitations beforehand?	Suggests arrhythmia (although fluttering in the stomach suggests temporal lobe epilepsy)
Did you have any chest pain or shortness of breath?	Suggests cardiorespiratory cause
Did you feel sweaty or sick beforehand?	May suggest hypoglycaemia but also can occur in cardiac, neurological and vestibular conditions
Did you notice any other strange sensations beforehand?	Visual or olfactory aura may suggest epilepsy; ringing in ears may indicate Ménière's disease.
Did you lose consciousness?	Often with cardiac syncope, patients improve once they hit the ground or lie down. Complete loss of consciousness suggests a neurological cause
Do you have any other medical conditions?	An essential question since many conditions are associated with syncope. Especially check for history of ischaemic heart disease, cerebrovascular disease and diabetes
What medications are you taking?	In particular, drugs that may cause hypoglycaemia, postural hypotension and arrhythmias
Does moving your head bring on these turns?	Suggests vertebro-basilar disease or benign positional vertigo
Do you notice the room spinning or ringing in your ears?	Suggestive of vestibular problem

Fact sheet: Features suggestive of epilepsy

If it is possible to get a witnessed account from an observer, it is important to ascertain whether this was an epileptiform attack or cardiac in nature. The following would make a diagnosis of epilepsy more likely.

- Tongue biting
- Incontinence
- Blue face (not pale)
- Loss of consciousness for more than 5 minutes
- Convulsive movements
- Disorientation on recovery for variable length of time

Pyrexia of unknown origin (PUO)

Dear Dr.
I would be grateful for your opinion on Mr. John Martin, a 42-year-old pharmacist. He presented to me a month ago with persistent fever with no obvious source. He has not responded to antibiotics.
Yours Sincerely

Dr. Hardwood

Essential skills required

- Knowledge of causes of pyrexia of unknown origin (PUO).
- Ability to take focussed history.

Think list

Your objectives	Mr. Martin's view
• Obtain clear focussed history.	• He has been unwell for a month and is fed up at the lack of progress.
• Identify most likely cause for PUO.	• He is self-employed and is worried that his business is beginning to suffer as he has been unable to work.

Danger! Common pitfalls

There are several common mistakes which students make that can be easily avoided.

✗ Lack of basic knowledge.
✗ Not allowing dialogue/allowing patient to ramble.
✗ Use of medical jargon.
✗ Insensitive approach to asking questions.

A PUO is defined as a prolonged fever for over 3 weeks, the cause of which has not been determined. Occasionally, the diagnosis can be very difficult, and in such cases it is vital to take a meticulously detailed history, concentrating on the possible causes outlined in fact sheet, page 160. It is also important to do a meticulous clinical examination, paying particular reference to the skin, looking for signs of vasculitis. If no diagnosis emerges, take the history again and repeat the clinical examination. It may well take several weeks to establish the diagnosis, and the patient needs to be advised of this at the outset.

Fact sheet: Essential questions in assessment of PUO	
Essential questions	*Clinical relevance*
Any associated symptoms?	• A full history of associated symptoms is essential to give clues to the cause of PUO • Joint pains suggest immunological cause • Weight loss may point to malignancy • Dyspnoea may suggest infection • Altered bowel habit may suggest inflammatory bowel disease
Exposure to any of the following?	
• Travel	See Chapter 20
• Medicines	See fact sheet, page 161
• Unusual foods	Unpasteurised milk suggests brucellosis
• Infected individuals	May give clues to pathogen
• Sexual contacts	May suggest HIV related illness
• Tattoos	May suggest blood-borne cause
• Recent surgery	Possibility of abscess
• Illicit drug use	Hepatitis, HIV-related
• Animal contact	Sick parrot suggest psittacosis
Does anyone else have the same problem?	
Vaccination history	
Previous psychiatric history	A significant proportion of PUOs are factitious. More common in healthcare workers

Fact sheet: Causes of a PUO

Cause	Commentary

Infection
• Deep-seated bacterial
  — subphrenic/perinephric abscess
  — osteomyelitis
• Infectious endocarditis (blood culture negative)
  — Q fever
  — aspergillus
• Granulomatous disease
  — TB
  — actinomycosis
  — histoplasmosis
  — toxoplasmosis
• Travellers
  — malaria
  — amoebiasis
  — schistosomiasis
• Non-localising infection
  — brucellosis
	• A search for a viral cause for PUO is likely to be unrewarding
	
	• Endocarditis caused by bacteria is usually blood culture +ve
	• An atrial myxoma can also cause a PUO
	• The CXR changes of military TB can occur several weeks into the disease
	
	• Full travel history is essential
	
	• Brucellosis usually has few localising symptoms or signs

Cancer • Lymphoma • Leukaemia • Sarcoma • Pancreas • Lung • Renal cell	• Lymphoproliferative neoplasia is the commonest cause of PUO in this category
Immunological • Rheumatic fever • Rheumatoid arthritis • Polyarteritis nodosa • Giant cell arteritis • Vasculitis • Still's disease	• The commonest cause in this category is a non-specific vasculitis • These conditions are usually very responsive to corticosteroid therapy, or other forms of immunosuppression

Fact sheet: Causes of a PUO—cont'd

Miscellaneous
- Sarcoidosis
- Crohn's
- Recurrent pulmonary emboli
- Chronic granulomatous hepatitis
- Drug fever
- CNS lesion affecting thermoregulation
- Factitious

Note: despite extensive and rigorous investigation the cause of PUO remains undetermined in approximately 10%.

Fact sheet: Drugs causing pyrexia

Antibiotics	Cardiac medicines	Miscellaneous
• Erythromycin • Isoniazid • Penicillin • Nitrofurantoin • Procainamide • Quinidine	• Atropine • Captopril • Hydralazine • Clofibrate • Nifedipine • Methyldopa • Hydrochlorothiazide	• Allopurinol • Antihistamines • Aspirin • Cimetidine • Heparin • Phenytoin

---

Fact sheet: Fever patterns in PUO

The pattern of fever rarely gives clues to the cause of pyrexia. However there are a few patterns worth remembering.

Malaria
- *Plasmodium falciparum*—temperature and rigors for 8–12 hours a day
- *Plasmodium vivax*—fevers every 48 hours with intervening apyrexia

Occult abscess
- High spiking fevers 39–40°C
- Usually above 37.5 in morning with evening peaks

Adult Stills disease
- Hectic fever with high peaks and a relative bradycardia

Hodgkin's
- Night sweats and fever

Fever on return from abroad

Lucy Mewes is a 22-year-old student who returned a week ago from a round-the-world trip. She presents with a 4-day history of intermittent fever and chills with documented temperatures of 39°C. Take a history to help establish possible causes.

Essential skills required

- Knowledge of causes of imported fever.
- Knowledge of public health issues regarding transmissible infections.
- Ability to take focussed history.

Think list

Your agenda
- Obtain clear focussed history.
- Identify possible cause of fever.
- Be aware of which infections are notifiable.
- Be aware of which infections are a public health concern.

Miss Mewes' agenda
- Wants to know what is wrong with her.
- Frustrated at the inconvenience of needing to go to the doctors.
- Might be scared that she has caught something serious.

Danger! Common pitfalls

There are several common mistakes which students make that can be easily avoided.

✗ Lack of basic knowledge.
✗ Not allowing dialogue/allowing her to ramble.
✗ Use of medical jargon.
✗ Insensitive approach to asking questions.

The best way to handle this scenario is to ask the patient to give you a history of her illness and then a travel history. You will get marks for allowing the patient to talk and demonstrating listening skills. It is acceptable to clarify things as you go along and may be necessary in order to keep the account focussed.

By allowing dialogue, you will hopefully obtain most of the information you require in the essential questions fact sheet (below). Once the patient has given her account, you can use some closed questions looking at specific points relevant to the history.

It is essential to ask questions sensitively. The temptation is to reel off a list of questions without considering the consequences of asking them. You will need to ask about sexual activities. This will not only be potentially embarrassing for the patient, but also highlights that you are considering sexually transmissible diseases, such as HIV.

Fact sheet: Essential questions in assessment of fever on return from abroad	
Essential questions	*Clinical relevance*
Where did you visit?	Is this a malaria region?
	What other diseases are endemic?
How long did you stay there?	Important when considering the incubation period of infections
Were you unwell at any time?	Take history of illness and treatment received to give clues to sources of infection
What vaccinations prior to travel?	• Vital to indicate infections protected against
	• Remember that malaria prophylaxis is only 70–90% effective and compliance is poor
	• Malaria prophylaxis does not exclude malaria
What medicines are you taking?	Drug history including immunosuppressants and recreational drugs
Was water local, bottled or sterilised?	Suggests enteric pathogens
Any unpasteurised dairy products?	Suggests brucellosis, enteric pathogens
Did you have sex whilst abroad?	Will need to take a full sexual history
	History should focus on acute HIV and other sexually transmitted infections
Any freshwater contact?	Suggests amoebiasis, schistosomiasis, leptospirosis
Animal contact?	Consideration of anthrax
Did any insects bite you?	Highly unlikely not to be bitten abroad but some bites may be memorable; dengue will result in a generalised rash
Any unusual activities?	Caving in America suggests histoplasmosis

Fact sheet: Infectious causes of fever following travel	
Tropical	
Common	• Malaria (N)
	• Acute viral hepatitis (N)*
	• Enteric fever (N)*
	• Dengue
	• Diarrhoeal illness
Less common	• Acute HIV infection*
	• Amoebic abscess
	• Rickettsial infection
	• Filiariasis
Essential to consider	• Viral haemorrhagic fever (N)*
Cosmopolitan	• Tuberculosis (N)*
	• Meningitis (N)*
	• Urinary tract infection
	• Respiratory infection
N, Notifiable disease. *Transmission is a public health issue.	

21

Shortness of breath

Mr. Geoffrey Roper, a 72-year-old retired builder, is referred to see you in clinic with breathlessness. Please take a structured history to determine the cause of this symptom.

Essential skills required

- Knowledge of differential diagnosis of breathlessness in a 72-year-old man.
- Generic history taking skills.

Think list

Your agenda
- Obtain clear focussed history.
- Determine cause of dyspnoea.
- Outline plan of investigation.
- Address hidden agenda.

Mr. Roper's agenda
- Scared he may have cancer.
- Breathlessness is affecting his quality of life.

Danger! Common pitfalls

✗ Lack of knowledge of differential diagnosis (fact sheets, p. 166 and p. 168).

✗ Not uncovering patient's agenda.

✗ Not taking an adequate smoking history. The smoking history should capture the amount of tobacco products consumed in the patient's lifetime, expressed in pack years.

✗ Not taking an adequate occupational history. This is very important in a patient with breathlessness, as some occupational diseases such as coalminer's pneumoconiosis will make the patient eligible for financial compensation. You also need to carefully document asbestos exposure (builders, car fitters, boiler-fitters, etc.), which is associated with asbestosis and mesothelioma for the same reason.

✗ Failure to determine the degree of functional impairment. You need to determine the amount of exercise the patient can perform before becoming breathless. This is usually best determined by the question 'how far can you walk on the flat without stopping?' If the breathlessness is due to heart failure apply the New York Heart Association classification (below).

New York Heart Association Classification	
Grade I	exercise tolerance uncompromised
Grade II	exercise tolerance slightly compromised
Grade III	exercise tolerance moderately compromised
Grade IV	exercise tolerance severely compromised

It is also important to establish at an early stage in the consultation whether the patient's breathlessness is acute in onset, or has come on in a more chronic indolent fashion. The reason for this is that the differential diagnosis of acute dyspnoea (onset in minutes or hours) is quite different to chronic dyspnoea (onset over days, months or years). Please see fact sheets below and on page 168.

Ask if there has been any haemoptysis associated with the breathlessness. There are a limited number of conditions that cause a combination of haemoptysis and breathlessness (fact sheet, p. 169).

Fact sheet: Causes of acute dyspnoea in a 72-year-old male	
Cause	*Symptoms*
Acute left ventricular failure	• Sudden onset of breathlessness (minutes to hours) • Often in the night • Patient has to sit up to ease dyspnoea • Associated with sweating, nausea and chest pain • May also have frothy white or pink-tinged sputum • May have past history of angina/MI
Pulmonary embolus	• Abrupt onset of breathlessness (seconds to minutes) • Associated with pleuritic chest pain usually (but not always) • Haemoptysis occurs in a minority • Clinical deep venous thrombosis is present only in a minority

Fact sheet: Causes of acute dyspnoea in a 72-year-old male—cont'd	
Cause	*Symptoms*
	• Check for risk factors — Past history of thromboembolism — Recent surgery — Recent immobilisation, e.g. international flight — Family history — Pro-thrombotic drugs, e.g. stilbestrol
Acute asthmatic attack	• Onset minutes to hours • Precipitated by cold weather and exercise • Associated wheeze • Usually have past history of similar attacks going back many years. Asthma occasionally presents at this age for the first time but this is uncommon
Chest infection	• Onset hours to days • Associated with cough and fever • Purulent or blood-stained sputum in a minority (cough is non-productive in many patients) • General malaise • Confusion is commonly found in this age-group, particularly with atypical (e.g. *Legionella* spp) or severe infections • Don't forget to ask if his budgie is off its food and has a runny beak! This would raise the possibility of psittacosis. This responds well to tetracycline if diagnosed early enough.
Pneumothorax	• Primary pneumothorax is very uncommon at this age • It is most commonly seen when a bulla 'pops' in a patient with chronic obstructive pulmonary disease/emphysema • It is usually associated with unilateral pleuritic pain • The diagnosis may be difficult as they are often small and easily missed on chest X-ray. The degree of breathlessness is usually out of proportion to the size of the pneumothorax seen on X-ray
Note: Do not forget that the age of the patient affects the differential diagnosis. For example, hyperventilation is a very common cause of breathlessness in a patient in the 20's but is extremely rare in a patient of this age.	

Fact sheet: Causes of chronic dyspnoea in a 72-year-old male	
Cause	*Symptoms*
Common causes	
Chronic obstructive pulmonary disease (COPD)	• Onset over months or years • May have chronic 'smokers' cough • Usually have a significant smoking history, but remember patients in their 70's and 80's can develop this condition without having smoked • Role of passive smoking • May have had numerous chest infections in the past necessitating hospital admission
Chronic asthma	• Usually there is a long history of attacks of breathlessness and wheeze, responding to bronchodilators • Asthma can start at this age but this is not common • Breathlessness is associated with wheeze and aggravated by cold weather and exercise • Symptoms often show a diurnal variation, with dips in peak flow readings in the morning
Chronic heart failure	• Onset over days, weeks or months • Breathlessness graded using New York Heart Association Classification • Patients have orthopnoea and paroxysmal nocturnal dyspnoea on a background of chronic breathlessness • May have peripheral oedema if both ventricles are failing • May have a past history of ischaemic or valvular heart disease.
Lung cancer	• Onset over days, weeks or months • May have associated haemoptysis, weight loss and cachexia • Smoking history, including history of passive smoking • Patients sometimes lose the taste for cigarettes when this disease develops
Pleural effusion	• Onset over weeks • Common causes include metastatic cancer and heart failure
Multiple pulmonary emboli	• Onset over weeks or months • May have episodes of acute breathlessness/ haemoptysis or syncope, but gradually increasing breathlessness is more common • Can be difficult to diagnose • May have symptoms of right heart failure, e.g. peripheral oedema

Fact sheet: Causes of chronic dyspnoea in a 72-year-old male—cont'd	
Cause	*Symptoms*
	• Check for risk factors for thromboembolic disease
Uncommon causes Fibrosing alveolitis Mesothelioma Asbestosis Pneumoconiosis Extrinsic allergic alveolitis Pericardial effusion	

Fact sheet: Dyspnoea with haemoptysis
• Carcinoma of the lung • Pulmonary tuberculosis • Pulmonary oedema, especially due to untreated mitral stenosis • Pulmonary embolism • Bacterial pneumonia, especially *Pneumococcus* • Bronchiectasis
Note: 1. Haemoptysis in bronchiectasis is rare but can be massive. 2. A cause for haemoptysis is frequently not found. These patients often have no associated dyspnoea.

22

Suicide risk

Jean Hayes is a 59-year-old unemployed lady, admitted via Accident and Emergency having taken an overdose. She is now medically fit for discharge. Take a focussed history to ascertain her suicide risk.

Essential skills required

- Knowledge of suicide risk and intent.
- Ability to discuss complex issues in a clear concise way.
- Use of non-medical jargon.
- Assess whether patient is likely to self-harm.

Think list

Your objectives	Miss Hayes' view
• Identify likelihood that she will attempt self-harm again. • Assess whether she is mentally unwell. • Ensure adequate support post discharge.	• It was all a big mistake, which she now regrets. • Doesn't want to talk at length about it.

Danger! Common pitfalls

There are several common mistakes which students make that can be easily avoided.

- ✗ Lack of basic knowledge.
- ✗ Unsympathetic approach.
- ✗ Use of medical jargon.
- ✗ Failure to deal with patient concerns.

One of the commonest presentations to the Accident and Emergency department are patients with deliberate self-harm (DSH). Many attend more than once and some will receive unsympathetic assessment and treatment. It is not our place to judge these unfortunate patients. Many have truly awful stories, are profoundly depressed and attempt to take their life as a last resort. There are others who use DSH as part of some broader manipulative behaviour. Your role is to take a history to assess whether DSH patients are safe to go home, i.e. are they likely to try and kill themselves if discharged. You are not just assessing suicidal intent, but also whether they are suffering from a mental illness. You will need to ascertain what support structure they have in place and make plans for safe follow-up.

It is important to note that not all DSH patients act with the intention of killing themselves. It is worth checking the patient's motivation for the attempt, since it may be for other reasons.

Reasons people self-harm

- To die
- To escape from unbearable anguish
- To get relief
- To change the behaviour of others
- To escape from a situation
- To show desperation to others
- To get back at other people/make them feel guilty
- To get help

As part of your assessment you need to identify the following:

- **Suicide intent,** i.e. the extent to which the patient wanted to harm herself. This gives you an indication as to how seriously the patient wanted to take his or her own life. Do not dismiss an overdose of non-toxic medicine as a low-intention attempt. The issue is whether the patient believed it would result in death. A patient eating a bag of peanuts doesn't sound suicidal until you discover he has a peanut allergy!
- **Suicide risk,** i.e. the likelihood that they will attempt to kill themselves again. This will help guide you in immediate and future psychiatric support.

Features that suggest a high suicidal intent are listed below.

High suicide intent

- Act carried out in isolation
- Act timed so that intervention unlikely
- Precautions taken to avoid discovery
- Preparations made in anticipation of death (e.g. making will, organising insurance)
- Preparations made for the act (e.g. purchasing means, saving up tablets)
- Communicating intent to others beforehand
- Leaving a note
- Not alerting potential helpers after the act

An easy way of remembering features suggestive of high suicide risk is by the mnemonic SAD PERSON (below).

High suicide risk (sad person)

- **S**ex: male > female
- **A**ge: more likely in older people
- **D**ivorced or separated
- **P**hysical illness, especially long-term poor health
- **E**mployment: higher risk in unemployed
- **R**ecurrent attempts
- **S**ocially isolated, living alone
- **O**ther mental illnesses, i.e. depression, alcoholism, schizophrenia
- **N**ote left, to explain the reasons for suicide

When interviewing a DSH patient, be empathic and show that you are listening. Do not become distressed by their distress. Do not be afraid to reflect frequently to encourage dialogue.

Do not worry about asking questions like 'Were you trying to kill yourself' or 'Are you suicidal'. Sometimes students worry that by using these words they may put the idea into the patient's head. This is not the case. Truly suicidal patients will not hide their intentions and will openly talk about it.

Thinking about suicide is not the same as suicidal intent. If a patient mentions that they feel suicidal or have thought about killing themselves, it is worth asking if they are planning to act on these thoughts. A person making active plans is much more of a worry than someone talking about it.

Fact sheet: Essential questions in assessment of patient at risk of suicide	
Essential questions	*Clinical relevance*
• Could you tell me a little about the events leading up to you coming into hospital?	Open question to allow dialogue. If patient is not keen to talk, you may need to use close questions earlier in the interview
• Has anything occurred recently that lead you to do this?	Try to identify precipitating life events
• Was this something you had planned or was it done on the spur of the moment? • Was anybody nearby who might have found you? • Did you write a suicide note? • Had you made any preparations for after you had gone?	Identify degree of pre-planning or whether this was an impulsive act. The following few questions are to assess the level of suicidal intent in the act. Actions, such as arranging for the dog to be put down, paying bills or writing a will, identify long-term planning and fixed, focussed intent
• Have you ever tried something like this before?	Higher likelihood of repeated attempts if there is a previous history
• Have you ever been treated for any medical or psychiatric conditions? • Do you drink much alcohol?	Higher risk of repeated attempts with chronic, disabling medical conditions, psychiatric illness and alcohol/drug abuse
• Does anyone live at home with you?	Social isolation; expand question to look at current support network
• How have you been sleeping recently?	Identify insomnia, panic attacks and poor memory; all suggesting depression
• Were you trying to kill yourself? • How do you feel about things now?	Was it the patient's intention to die? Will the patient do it again?

23

Taking an alcohol history

A 25-year-old pharmaceutical representative attends her family doctor as she fell down the stairs the previous night and badly bruised her ribs. She would like a sick note. This has happened to her twice before in the last 3 years.

Take a history from this patient to determine the cause of her problem.

Essential skills required

- Knowledge of causes of falls in a 25-year-old female.
- Ability to take an accurate alcohol history.
- Generic history taking skills.

Think list

Your agenda	Mrs. Farmer's agenda
• Obtain clear focussed history.	• To obtain a sick note.
• Determine cause of falls.	• To avoid discussing her
• Take an accurate alcohol history.	alcohol intake if at all possible.

Danger! Common pitfalls

✗ Lack of basic knowledge.
✗ Insensitive approach.
✗ Not identifying alcohol as the most likely cause of her falls.

The CAGE questionnaire is a useful tool that can be employed to identify patients with alcohol misuse.

CAGE questionnaire for alcohol misuse
• Have you ever felt you ought to **C**ut down on your drinking? • Have people **A**nnoyed you by criticising your drinking? • Have you ever felt **G**uilty about your drinking? • Have you ever needed a drink first thing in the morning to steady your nerves or get rid of a hangover (**E**ye-opener)?
Note: Two or more positive replies are said to identify problem drinkers.

Taking an alcohol history

To take a complete alcohol history you need to determine the amount of alcohol currently consumed. It is also essential to determine the amount of alcohol consumed in the recent and distant past. To achieve this you need to know the alcohol content of common beverages.

Alcohol content of common beverages
• $^1/_2$ pint beer = 1 unit • 1 small glass of table wine = 1 unit • 1 pub measure of spirits = 1 unit • 1 bottle wine = 6–7 units • 1 standard bottle of spirits = 32 units

When you determine the quantity of alcohol consumed by the patient, remember that patients will commonly underestimate the amount consumed by up to 100%. You need to determine the patient's current drinking habits in terms of the frequency of alcohol consumption, types of drinks consumed and the quantity of each alcoholic beverage consumed in order to come up with a weekly total at the end. Remember to check whether the patient drinks in the morning or at lunchtime. Remember also that there is a vast difference between pub measures of drinks and drinks taken at home. This is often a major source of error in estimating the quantity of alcohol consumed. One of the ways to get round this is to ask how long a bottle of spirits would last.

Another source of underestimation of alcohol consumption is accurately determining the type of alcohol drunk and knowing the alcohol content of the drink taken (see above table). For example, the alcohol content of special brew lager can be up to four times that of standard lager.

The current recommendations for safe alcohol consumption are 21 units/week for men and 14 units/week for women. There are a number of professions who are at high risk of alcohol abuse and these include:

- armed forces
- merchant seamen
- publicans
- entertainment industry
- doctors.

Patients with an alcohol problem only infrequently present to a doctor and say 'Doctor, I think I am an alcoholic. Can you help me please?' More commonly they present with a complication of their alcohol abuse. These are summarised in the fact sheet below. Therefore, when you encounter any of these conditions it is mandatory to take a full and accurate alcohol history.

Fact sheet: Common presentations of alcohol abuse

- Fits—commonly seen on alcohol withdrawal
- Delirium tremens—agitation, confusion, sweating and hallucinations. Commonly seen on alcohol withdrawal
- Falls/trauma—broken ribs are common in alcoholics who tend to fall over when inebriated. Head injury is also common
- Road traffic accidents—caused by driving whilst under the influence of alcohol
- Acute pancreatitis—an alcoholic binge is one of the commonest causes (along with gallstone disease) of acute pancreatitis. This condition can be severe and life-threatening and may require management in the intensive care unit
- Decompensation of chronic ethanolic liver disease:
  — bleeding oesophageal varices
  — jaundice due to alcoholic hepatitis
  — ascites
  — hepatic encephalopathy
- Pulmonary tuberculosis, chest infections and aspiration pneumonia
- Alcoholic cardiomyopathy
- Wernicke–Korsakoff syndrome
- Peripheral neuropathy—glove and stocking and usually predominantly sensory

---

24

Weight loss

A 72-year-old man is referred to you with weight loss. Take a structured history from this patient and construct a differential diagnosis.

Essential skills required

- Knowledge of differential diagnosis of weight loss in a 72-year-old man (see fact sheet, p. 178).
- Generic consultation skills.

Think list

Doctor's agenda
- Take an accurate weight loss history (fact sheets, pp. 178–180)
- Knowledge of differential diagnosis of weight loss (fact sheet, p. 178).

Patient's agenda
- Patient is not sure why he has lost weight.
- May be worried he has cancer.

Danger! Common pitfalls

✘ Lack of knowledge.
✘ Not taking into account the patients age and sex. For example, anorexia nervosa or thyrotoxicosis should not really figure in the differential diagnosis of weight loss in a 72-year-old man, but should do in a 20-year-old woman.
✘ Ignoring possible diagnosis of depression.

You need to be very careful about the diagnosis of depression as the cause of an elderly patient's weight loss. In fact, depression is a common cause of weight loss in the elderly, but this diagnosis often has to be made by excluding the other causes of weight loss detailed in the fact sheet, page 178.

Fact sheet: Causes of weight loss
Diet   • Reducing diet   • Iatrogenic, e.g. fat free diet for gallstones   • Protein–calorie malnutrition
Anorexia nervosa
Depression
Bereavement
Increased exercise
Reduced appetite   • Peptic ulcer   • Stomach cancer   • Post gastropexy   • Iatrogenic, e.g. digoxin toxicity
Malabsorption   • Coeliac disease   • Crohn's disease
Chronic disorders   • Tuberculosis   • Vasculitis   • Crohn's disease

Cancer
 • Metastatic
 • Organ specific
   • Lung
   • Oesophagus
   • Stomach
   • Lymphoma

Metabolic   • Diabetes mellitus   • Thyrotoxicosis
Cardiac   • End-stage cardiac failure 'cardiac cachexia'
Idiopathic

Fact sheet: Essential features of a weight loss history

It is important to establish the following in a patient who has lost weight:

How much weight have you lost?
A weight loss of 1–2 kg is very common and often relates to small changes in diet or exercise. Weight loss of greater than 3 kg is more significant.

Over what time period has the weight loss occurred?
Significant weight loss over a short period of time increases the chance of there being an organic explanation for the weight loss.

Whether weight loss is progressive or not
Rapid and progressive weight loss is common in patients with the cancers detailed in the fact sheet above. It is also occasionally seen in other conditions, e.g. new onset diabetes, vasculitis, and Crohn's disease.

Whether the weight loss was deliberate
The commonest cause of weight loss is that the patient is on a reducing diet. Don't forget that prescribed diets can also cause a patient to lose weight, e.g. a patient with gallstones who is put on a fat-free diet will invariably lose weight.

Past history of episodes of weight loss
Weight in some patients seems to 'yo-yo' by 3–4 kg. The reason for this is not clear. Many patients say they lose weight in the summer and this may relate to changes in diet and exercise. Patients with anorexia nervosa have often had multiple episodes of significant weight loss in the past.

Any other associated symptoms?
See fact sheet below.

Fact sheet: Associated symptoms in weight loss

When taking a history from a patient with weight loss you need to ask some specific questions regarding associated symptoms, bearing the differential diagnosis in mind (fact sheet, p. 178). These include:

Anorexia nervosa
This is a common problem. 95% of patients are in their teens or 20's and are female. They often have had several bouts of weight loss in the past and may have a psychiatric history as well. Some patients will admit to self-induced vomiting. Nearly all patients have a distorted self body image. This can usually be uncovered by asking the patient what she thinks her ideal weight should be. Anorexics are frequently less than frank when giving a history, and it is important to try to ascertain corroboratory evidence from the patient's family and or family doctor.

Depression
This is a common cause of weight loss, particularly in the middle-aged and elderly. It can be a difficult diagnosis to make, and in patients with

---

Fact sheet: Associated symptoms in weight loss—cont'd

profound weight loss it is important to ensure that a physical cause for the weight loss is excluded first. Patients often have associated sleep disturbance (early morning waking), low mood with diurnal variation (worse in the mornings). There may be a history of a recent major life-event, e.g. bereavement.

Bereavement
Bereaved patients very commonly lose weight due to a combination of depression and a change in diet.

Peptic ulcer
Patients usually have associated epigastric discomfort related to meals, anorexia and or nausea.

Iatrogenic
Drugs can cause weight loss in some patients and a full drug history is essential. For example, digoxin toxicity causes anorexia, nausea, and disturbed taste. Patients may also complain of a visual disturbance with objects taking on a slight yellow hue.

Crohn's disease
Patients will almost invariably have recurrent abdominal pain and diarrhoea. This may be relatively longstanding (years). Systemic symptoms such as mouth ulceration, iritis and arthralgia occur in about 50%.

Pulmonary tuberculosis
Chronic cough and haemoptysis in a patient from a high-risk group (IVDU, refugees, alcoholics, immigrants from SE Asia).

Cancer
- Metastatic—malaise, anorexia
- Lung—cough, haemoptysis, breathlessness, smoking history
- Oesophagus—progressive dysphagia

25

Tired all the time

Mrs. Gillian Ramsbottom, a 46-year-old housewife, comes to see you complaining of being tired all the time. Take a history from her to try to elucidate the cause.

Essential skills required

- Knowledge of differential diagnosis of fatigue in a 46-year-old woman.
- Generic consultation skills.

Think list

Your agenda
- Exclude organic cause for symptoms.
- Identify precipitant for presentation.
- Address any questions or anxieties.

Mrs. Ramsbottom's agenda
- Worried there is something seriously wrong with her.

Danger! Common pitfalls

There are several common mistakes which students make that can be easily avoided.

✗ Not checking current understanding and concerns.
✗ Poor listening skills.
✗ Failing to exclude organic causes.

'Tired all the time' is a very common symptom in general practice. It is important to ensure that the patient does not have organic disease first (see fact sheet, pp. 182, 184). However, in 95% of patients consulting their family doctor with this symptom, no organic cause will be found. Often patients will not accept this or, at best, reluctantly do so. It is vital that you take the patient's symptoms seriously. You need to be quite clear to the patient that, although there may be no physical explanation for the symptoms, this does not mean that the patient is either mad or malingering. If you do not achieve this, the relationship between you and the patient may be irrevocably damaged. This may have a negative effect on the patient's ability to come to terms with the problem and may delay or impede recovery.

Remember that at any one time, 20–30% of the population will feel fatigued. Fatigue is a very subjective symptom. It is quite impossible to measure the degree of fatigue in an every day setting in the clinic or practice surgery. The commonest cause is overwork or lack of sleep, and these areas should be the first port of call when taking the history.

A detailed history, with a complete systems review, is necessary in any patient who presents with fatigue. The reason for this is that fatigue is a symptom that is found in many diseases (see fact sheet below). It is, therefore, important to exclude these as far as possible by taking a detailed history. However, when there is an organic cause for the patient's symptoms there are almost invariably other symptoms that point to the diagnosis. It is unusual for organic disease to present with the symptom of 'tired all the time' in isolation. For example, fatigue is a common symptom of new onset diabetes mellitus, but most patients with this condition will also have polyuria and polydypsia.

Having looked at the fact sheets on pages 182 and 184, it is clear that possible causes of tiredness are vast and beyond the scope of a single consultation. It is likely, therefore, that the scenario will point fairly clearly to either:

• organic cause/physical cause
• psychological/psychiatric cause
• chronic fatigue syndrome.

You will need to be flexible and focus the consultation appropriately. The fact sheet on page 184 gives a few questions that should be included in all consultations to ensure organic and non-organic causes are considered.

Fact sheet: Physical causes of fatigue	
Cause	Associated symptoms
Social • Overwork • Lack of sleep	

Fact sheet: Physical causes of fatigue—cont'd	
Cause	*Associated symptoms*
Cancer Lymphoma Leukaemia Carcinoma of the lung Carcinoma of the pancreas Metastatic disease	• Weight loss • Fever/sweats • Anorexia
Haematological Vasculitis RA Polyarteritis nodosa Mixed connective tissue disease	• Arthralgia • Rashes • Fever
Anaemia	• Breathlessness • Ankle oedema • Blood loss • GI symptoms
Endocrinological Diabetes mellitus Hypothyroidism Hyperthyroidism Addison's disease	• Polyuria, polydypsia, weight loss • Weight gain, feels the cold, rough skin • Weight loss, anxiety, tremor, diarrhoea • Skin pigmentation
Respiratory Chronic obstructive airways disease Carcinoma of the lung Tuberculosis	• Dyspnoea • Weight loss • Haemoptysis
Cardiac Infective endocarditis End stage heart failure Constrictive pericarditis	• Fever • Dyspnoea • Peripheral oedema
Renal failure	
Neurological Myasthenia gravis	• Easy fatigability • Diplopia
Iatrogenic Tricyclic antidepressants	• A full drug history is mandatory; remember that many hypnotic drugs have a hang-over effect, particularly in the elderly

Fact sheet: Non-physical causes of fatigue

Cause	Associated symptoms
Depression	• Low mood • Worse in morning • Early morning waking • Lack of sex drive • Suicidal ideation • Weight loss
Bipolar disorder	• Symptoms as above • Patients have manic phases which may last weeks or months
Poor sleep pattern	• Depression • Alcohol abuse • Idiopathic • Various physical causes, e.g. obstructive sleep apnoea, nocturia
Somatisation syndrome	• Fatigue is a prominent symptom in over 30% • Patients have an array of other physical symptoms with no organic explanation • Commoner in females • Patients have often had multiple negative invasive investigations or surgical procedures
Chronic fatigue syndrome	• See fact sheet on page 185

Fact sheet: Essential questions in assessment of chronic fatigue

Essential questions	Clinical relevance
I understand you have been feeling tired. Could you tell me a little about it?	Once again, start with an open question and allow dialogue. You may then focus on particular diagnoses with more closed questioning
Could you tell me a little about your sleep pattern?	Important to know whether they are getting sufficient restful sleep. Insomnia or early morning waking may suggest a non-organic cause
Do you feel rested after sleep?	May give clues to aetiology
What medications are you taking?	In particular ask about sedatives, hypnotics, anti-epileptics and painkillers

Fact sheet: Essential questions in assessment of chronic fatigue—cont'd	
Essential questions	Clinical relevance
Do you have any other medical conditions?	Tiredness may be a sign that these other conditions have altered
Have you noticed any change in your weight?	Weight loss may indicate organic pathology (but not exclusively); weight gain may suggest hypothyroidism
Have you noticed any other symptoms?	Systems review to check for diabetes, anaemia, etc.
Is there anything in particular that you think might be the cause of your tiredness?	Important to acknowledge and address their agenda

Chronic fatigue syndrome

This is also known as post-viral fatigue syndrome or ME. It is a commonly used diagnostic label in patients who have fatigue for which no cause has been determined. The prevalence is 0.2–2.6%. Diagnostic criteria have been drawn up, which are used mostly in research of this condition rather than in everyday clinical practice.

Fact sheet: CDC diagnostic criteria for chronic fatigue syndrome (1994)
• Fatigue with no explanation for >6 months
— New onset
— Not a result of on-going exertion
— Not relieved by rest
— Significant reduction in previous levels of activity
• Plus four or more of
— Subjective memory impairment
— Tender lymph nodes
— Muscle pain
— Joint pain
— Headache
— Un-refreshing sleep
— Post-exertion malaise (>24 hours)
• Exclusions
— Active, unresolved or suspected physical disease
— Psychotic disorders (not major depression)
— Dementia
— Anorexia/bulimia
— Alcohol abuse
— Severe obesity

In addition to the above diagnostic criteria, there are a number of important points to bear in mind when taking a history from a patient with chronic fatigue syndrome. This syndrome often follows a viral-type illness, but in most patients viral serological testing is negative. It is more common in females (M : F ratio is 1 : 1.7). Prognosis is better in children and in patients with an abrupt onset of symptoms. About 20–50% of patients show some improvement in the medium term, but only 6% achieve pre-morbid level of function.

Depressive symptoms are common in this group of patients and should be treated if found. However, antidepressant therapy has no effect on the final prognosis. Many other treatments have been tried including corticosteroids, graded exercise, prolonged rest and immunotherapy with immunoglobulins. All of these have no proven benefit and may do harm. The only therapy that has been shown to be beneficial is cognitive behaviour therapy.

26

Haematuria

Mr. Len Gooch is a 22-year-old man who attended for an insurance medical. He is found to have a positive urine dipstick for blood. Take a history to identify possible causes.

Essential skills required

- Knowledge of causes of haematuria and ability to differentiate between them.
- Ability to obtain relevant information.
- Focussed approach.
- Identify and deal with potentially serious causes of haematuria.

Think list

Your agenda
- Obtain clear focussed history.
- Identify serious causes of haematuria.
- Address any questions or anxieties.

Mr. Gooch's agenda
- Annoyed that this may prevent him getting insurance for a mortgage.
- Concerned that this may be something serious.

Danger! Common pitfalls

There are several common mistakes which students make that can be easily avoided.

✗ Not checking prior understanding.
✗ Lack of basic knowledge.
✗ Unsystematic approach.
✗ Ignoring Mr. Gooch's agenda.

The fact sheet on page 188 outlines causes of haematuria. Since this patient is young, the most likely cause is glomerular in origin. Tumours are rare in this age group but should be high on the differential in an older patient. Patients with haematuria are usually asymptomatic and so it is important to ask closed questions to focus on the likely causes.

It is important to anticipate that Mr. Gooch will be very unhappy about the dipstick finding. His insurance will be rejected until serious disease is ruled out and this may delay him getting a house. In the exam, the patient may be angry and not keen to give you any answers that he feels may jeopardise his chances of getting a mortgage.

Make sure you acknowledge his concerns and are prepared to listen to him vent his anger. Your role here is to allow him to express his anger but also to explain the importance of investigating his haematuria.

Once again the importance of checking prior understanding is important. At face value, Mr. Gooch may appear angry because the discovery of haematuria is slowing down his insurance application. However, his anger may be his way of expressing concern that something serious is going on. Since malignancy is an uncommon cause of haematuria in a man of this age, it would be reasonable to reassure him at this stage that cancer is an unlikely cause. Nevertheless, it is important to stress that other causes of haematuria, such as kidney disease, may be responsible, hence the importance of taking the dipstick findings seriously.

Fact sheet: Causes of haematuria

Renal blood loss	*Bladder/urinary tract blood loss*
• Glomerulonephritis — IgA nephropathy • Adult polycystic kidney disease • Tumours • Trauma	• Urinary stones • Tumours • Prostatic disease

---

Fact sheet: Likely investigations for haematuria

It is important to familiarise yourself with investigations that the patient may need and to be able to explain how they are carried out.

- Electrolytes
- Urine microscopy
- Blood pressure
- Plain radiograph: KUB to look for stones
- Ultrasound of renal tract: check size of kidneys, look for masses in kidney and bladder wall

If stones are a possibility:

- IVU

If glomerular disease suspected:

- Renal biopsy

In older patient:

- Cystoscopy

Fact sheet: Essential questions in assessment of haematuria

Essential questions	Clinical relevance
• Have you noticed any blood in the urine?	Frank haematuria occurs with stones and tumours, and if followed by microscopic haematuria suggests IgA nephropathy
• Have you noticed any back or loin pain?	Pain may suggest stones, polycystic kidney disease, infection or tumour Painless haematuria is more suggestive of glomerulonephritis, interstitial nephritis and possibly tumours
• Have you had a sore throat or infection recently?	As in post-infective glomerulonephritis
• Any increased urinary frequency or pain on passing water?	Suggests urinary tract infection
• Any joint pains or rashes?	If so consider multisystem disorder such as systemic vasculitis
• Have you passed any stones or grit in your water?	Points to renal stone disease
• Have you been doing heavy exercise or had an injury recently?	Trauma
• Have you been abroad recently?	Ask about travel to where *Schistosoma haematobium* is prevalent; infection may cause urinary tract granuloma and tumour formation
• What medicines are you taking? Have you taken any other medicines recently?	Drug history is essential; ask specifically about analgesics that may cause papillary necrosis
• Are there any illnesses that run in the family?	Polycystic kidney disease, Alport's syndrome.

Fact sheet: Basic information about IgA nephopathy

- IgA nephropathy is a kidney disorder caused by deposits of the protein immunoglobulin A (IgA) inside the glomeruli within the kidney.
- These glomeruli normally filter waste and excess water from the blood and send them to the bladder as urine.
- The IgA protein prevents this filtering process, leading to blood and protein in the urine and swelling in the hands and feet.
- It usually presents in males in their late teens or twenties and is often asymptomatic.
- This chronic kidney disease may progress over a period of 10–20 years.

Fact sheet: Basic information about IgA nephopathy—cont'd

- If this disorder leads to end-stage renal disease, the patient must go on dialysis or receive a kidney transplant. However, this only occurs in a small proportion of patients.
- The IgA protein, an antibody, is a normal part of the body's immune system, the system that protects against disease. We do not know what causes IgA deposits in the glomeruli but, since IgA nephropathy may run in families, genetic factors probably contribute to the disease.
- Kidney disease usually cannot be cured. Once the tiny filtering units are damaged, they cannot be repaired.
- Treatment focuses on slowing the progression of the disease and preventing complications. One complication is high blood pressure, which further damages glomeruli.
- A class of medicines called ACE inhibitors protects kidney function not only by lowering blood pressure but also by reducing the loss of protein into the urine.
- Patients with IgA nephropathy often have high cholesterol. Reducing cholesterol—through diet, medication, or both—appears to help slow the progression of IgA nephropathy.
- Corticosteroids may suppress the production of IgA.

27

Occupational illness

It is becoming more frequent to ask students to take an occupational history at some part of their exam. As with a sexual history, it is unlikely that you will be asked to take just an occupational history. It is more likely that you will need to include it somewhere in a scenario. The most common example is:

Mr. Nick Fairman, aged 64, presents to his GP with dyspnoea and cough. His chest X-ray shows pleural thickening with a right pleural effusion. Take a focussed history from him.

Essential skills required

- Ability to take an occupational history.
- Sensitive approach.
- Anticipate patient anxieties concerning diagnosis.
- Be aware of medico-legal aspects of occupational disease.

Think list

Your agenda	Mr. Fairman's agenda
• Obtain clear focussed history.	• Scared he has cancer.
• Identify if there is any occupational cause for lung disease.	• May or may not be aware that his illness could be related to previous employment.
• Address any questions or anxieties.	

Danger! Common pitfalls

There are several common mistakes which students make that can be easily avoided.

✗ Not checking prior understanding.
✗ Lack of basic knowledge.
✗ Insensitive approach.
✗ Ignoring Mr. Fairman's anxieties.

Pleural thickening is commonly associated with asbestos-related lung disease, as listed in the fact sheet below. In this particular scenario, candidates would be expected to include a full occupational history to identify exposure. In addition, they may need to discuss the possible diagnosis and be prepared to break bad news if malignancy is a possibility.

Fact sheet: Essential questions to assess asbestos exposure	
Essential questions	*Clinical relevance*
• It is important for me to know about the jobs you have done in the past, even those from many years ago. It would be helpful if you could go through the jobs you have done since leaving school.	Although laborious, this method is more systematic and likely to identify all jobs he has done It is important to establish what he did in each job
• Do you remember at any time working with asbestos?	Having asked an open question, try a closed question to ascertain exposure. Do not forget to ask about holiday jobs. Even exposure 40 years ago is significant
If answer is yes, ask the following questions.	
— For how long in the day were you in contact?	Gives an idea of exposure
— Did you have protective clothing or masks?	Check whether employers provided these, as there may be compensation issues
— Were your clothes covered in asbestos dust?	Further indication of severity of exposure
If answer is no, include the following questions.	
— Did anyone in your family work with asbestos? — If so did they come home with dust on their clothes?	Further clues to exposure
— How much do you smoke?	Important to know how much and for how long since it will have legal implications

---

Fact sheet: Presentations associated with asbestos exposure

Common	Less common
• Pleural thickening	• Asbestosis
• Pleural plaques	• Lung cancer
	• Mesothelioma

Fact sheet: Taking an occupational history

Essential questions	Clinical relevance
• Tell me a little about your symptoms.	A good open-ended question. If necessary focus on any system affected. Try and find out what the patient attributes the symptoms to
• Are your symptoms different at work and at home?	Symptoms exacerbated at work may suggest occupational exposure
• Do any of your co-workers have similar symptoms?	If so it makes occupational illness much more likely
• It is important for me to know about the jobs you have done in the past, even those from many years ago. It would be helpful if you could go through the jobs you have done since leaving school.	As stated before a detailed occupational history is essential and must include tasks done in the job and not just job title
• Ask about exposure to:	
— Chemicals (e.g. formaldehyde, organic solvents, pesticides)	*Formaldehyde*—throat and nasal cancer *Organic solvents*—neurotoxicity *Pesticides*—neurotoxicity, prostate cancer
— Metals (e.g. lead, arsenic)	*Lead*—neurotoxic, abdominal pain *Arsenic*—lung and skin cancer
— Dusts (e.g. asbestos, silica, coal)	*Asbestos*—lung cancer, mesothelioma, etc. *Silica*—silicosis *Coal*—chronic lung disease
— Biological (e.g. HIV, hepatitis B, tuberculosis)	Self-explanatory
— Physical (e.g. noise, repetitive motion, radiation)	*Noise*—deafness *Repetitive strain injury* *Radiation*—cancer, thyroid problems, pulmonary fibrosis
— Psychological (e.g. stress)	*Stress*—depression, anxiety, post-traumatic stress disorder

Nocturnal cough

Dear Dr.
I would be grateful for your opinion on Mrs. Julia Wanford, a 52-year-old dinner lady who gives a three-month history of persistent nocturnal cough.
Yours Sincerely,

Dr. Yoreth

Take a focussed history from Mrs. Wanford. You do not need to examine her.

Essential skills required

- Knowledge of nocturnal cough.
- Ability to obtain relevant information.
- Empathic approach.
- Anticipate and manage Mrs.Wanford's concerns and questions.

Think list

Your agenda
- Obtain clear focussed history.
- Diagnose or rule out serious pathology.
- Address any questions or anxieties.

Mrs. Wanford's agenda
- May be worried she has cancer.
- May think referral to a specialist suggests something really *is* wrong.
- Cough is disturbing both her and her husband's sleep.

Danger! Common pitfalls

There are several common mistakes which students make that can be easily avoided.

✗ Lack of basic knowledge.
✗ Not checking current understanding.

✗ Use of medical jargon.
✗ Not acknowledging her concerns.

Chronic cough is defined as a cough lasting more than 3 weeks. The most common cause is smoking. It is important that you do not attribute all their symptoms to smoking since many of the other pathologies listed in the fact sheet on page 196 may occur in smokers. Often patients will be worried that they have cancer. It is important that you acknowledge their concerns but do not reassure them too much until you have ruled malignancy out.

Doctor:	Is there anything in particular you're concerned the cough may be due to?
Mrs. Wanford:	Yes doctor. I am terrified that I have got cancer.
Doctor:	Don't worry. I'm sure it isn't cancer. I promise.

Telling someone that they have cancer is hard enough. Delivering this news to someone that you have assured does not have cancer is even harder. Imagine how unexpected the news will be. They will be livid! It is much better to acknowledge their anxieties but not make false promises. Reflection can often help clarify their concerns before addressing the issues.

Doctor:	Is there anything in particular you're concerned the cough may be due to?
Mrs. Wanford:	Yes doctor. I am terrified that I have got cancer.
Doctor:	It sounds like you have been worrying about this for some time.
Mrs. Wanford:	Well, a neighbour of mine died of lung cancer and his started with a bad cough.
Doctor:	I can understand why you are so worried. *(pause)* There are many causes of a cough. *(pause)* Most of them are nothing to worry about. *(pause)* Cancer is one of the rarer causes and it is important that we rule this out so we can reassure you. *(pause)* I can't promise that you don't have cancer, but I think there are other causes that are more likely. What is important is that we do some tests to find out exactly what is happening.
Mrs. Wanford:	Okay doctor.

Fact sheet: Causes of cough

Productive	Non-productive
• Smoking	• Smoking
• Chronic bronchitis	• Asthma
• Chronic obstructive airways disease	• Postnasal drip
• Asthma	• Oesophageal reflux
• Bronchiectasis	• Drugs, e.g. ACE inhibitors
• Lung cancer	• Sarcoid
• Tuberculosis	• Connective tissue disease
• Congestive cardiac failure	• Congestive cardiac failure

Fact sheet: Essential questions in the assessment of nocturnal cough

Essential questions	Clinical relevance
• I understand you have been troubled by a cough. Tell me a little about it.	Begin with open question to allow dialogue and demonstrate listening skills
• When did it start?	Identify how long this has been going on and if there are any precipitants. Did anything else occur at the same time that may be associated, e.g. illness or change of medication?
• Do you cough up any muck?	Productive or non-productive cough may help to narrow down differential diagnosis
• Was it associated with a viral illness?	May suggest precipitants
• Have you had any problems with wheezing?	Often asthma first presents as nocturnal cough
• Do you ever get short of breath at night?	Consider chronic lung disease, congestive cardiac failure
• Do you have any medical illnesses?	May signify progression or loss of control of pre-existing condition
• Have you ever had problems with heartburn or indigestion?	Gastro-oesophageal reflux is often asymptomatic. Past history of peptic ulceration may give clues
• What medications are you taking?	Clues to underlying illnesses and check for ACE inhibitors
• How much do you smoke?	Smoking history essential
• Have you noticed any change in your weight?	Weight loss may suggest underlying malignancy although this can occur with many chronic illnesses

29

Acromegaly

Dear Dr.

I would be grateful if you would see Mr. Peter Stevens, a 45-year-old gardener who I think might have acromegaly.

Yours Sincerely,

Dr. Query

Take a focussed history from Mr. Stevens. You are not required to examine him.

Essential skills required

- Knowledge of clinical features of acromegaly and how it may present.
- Ability to obtain relevant information.
- Use of non-medical jargon.
- Anticipate and manage Mr. Stevens concerns and questions.

Think list

Your objectives	Mr. Stevens' view
• Obtain clear focussed history.	• May not understand what he's been referred for.
• Identify extent of disease if acromegaly is likely.	• May have noticed changes and is worried by them.
• Explain follow-up plans.	

Danger! Common pitfalls

There are several common mistakes which students make that can be easily avoided.

✗ Lack of basic knowledge.
✗ Not checking current understanding.
✗ Use of medical jargon.
✗ Insensitive approach to asking questions.

The clinical features of acromegaly are covered in *Final MB: A Guide to Success in Clinical Medicine*. You will recall that acromegaly is caused by an excess of growth hormone from a pituitary tumour. Your history should assess for physical changes and also for abnormal activity of pituitary hormones.

Patients may be aware that their physical appearance has changed and could well be embarrassed by this. Be careful to ask sensitive open questions before focussing on closed questions.

Fact sheet: Essential questions in assessing possible acromegaly	
Essential questions	*Clinical relevance*
• Have you noticed any headaches or problems with your vision?	These imply local tumour expansion. The classic visual disturbance is of bitemporal hemianopia
• Have you noticed any changes in your shoe size?	These questions pertain to growth hormone excess. You should check for altered facial features, snoring, arthralgia and cardiac failure. If possible ask the patient if they have any photos from a few years ago, to compare.
• Sometimes people notice that their facial features change. Have you been aware of anything like this?	
• Has anyone noticed that you are snoring more than usual?	Sweating is an important feature as it suggests continued growth hormone activity
• Have you noticed that you are sweating more than normal?	It is then important to check for evidence of pituitary dysfunction by asking questions about the various pituitary hormones
• Any joint pains or breathlessness?	
• Have there been any changes in your energy levels?	Tiredness may suggest ACTH deficiency or hypercapnia from sleep apnoea
• Have you noticed any change in your weight?	Weight gain with lethargy may suggest hypothyroidism
• Have you noticed any change in your sex drive?	Reduced libido, difficulties achieving/maintaining an erection may be due to hypogonadism. It is also worth asking about galactorrhoea, which may imply hyperprolactinaemia.
• Has anyone in the family had any hormone problems?	Although this may provoke a response about grandma's menopause, it is worth following on with a more closed question to check for a family history of hypercalcaemia. This may suggest multiple endocrine neoplasia type 1

30

Haematemesis

Mr. Larry Broadhead is a 63-year-old man who is admitted to hospital as an emergency with a haematemesis. Take a history to identify possible causes.

Essential skills required

- Knowledge of causes of haematemesis and ability to differentiate between them.
- Ability to obtain relevant information.
- Focussed approach.
- Identify and deal with potentially serious causes of haematemesis.

Think list

Your agenda
- Obtain clear focussed history.
- Identify serious causes of haematemesis.
- Address any questions or anxieties.

Mr. Broadhead's agenda
- Concerned that this may be something serious.

Danger! Common pitfalls

There are several common mistakes which students make that can be easily avoided.

- ✘ Not checking prior understanding.
- ✘ Lack of basic knowledge.
- ✘ Unsystematic approach.
- ✘ Ignoring Mr. Broadhead's agenda.

The fact sheet on page 200 outlines causes of haematemesis. Remember that in 40% of patients referred for an upper gastro-intestinal endoscopy with haematemesis, no cause is found.

Since haematemesis is a potentially life-threatening medical emergency, it is reasonable to state that you would first like to establish that the patient was haemodynamically stable and didn't require resuscitating. You would look a little silly if you tried to take a history from someone who was moribund from extensive blood loss! Although this is unlikely, it is possible that the examiner will ask how you would manage an acute haematemesis as part of a mini viva.

Do not forget that you may be required to discuss possible investigations for haematemesis such as an endoscopy. This is covered earlier in the book.

Fact sheet: Causes of haematemesis

Oesophageal	*Gastro-duodenal*
• Mallory–Weiss tear • Oesophageal varices • Oesophageal ulcer • Reflux oesophagitis • Oesophageal ulcer • Oesophageal cancer	• Peptic ulceration • Stomach cancer • Severe gastritis

---

Fact sheet: Essential questions in the assessment of haematemesis

Essential questions	*Clinical relevance*
• Tell me what has been happening to you.	Nice open question to start with
• What colour was the vomit?	Bright red indicates fresh bleeding, dark brown 'coffee grounds' indicates bleeding some time ago as the blood has been partially digested
• Did the blood appear the first time you vomited?	In a Mallory–Weiss tear the patient typically produces some bright red blood following one or previous episodes of vomiting normal gastric contents
• What quantity of blood did you vomit?	Patients find this difficult to quantify, and you may need to prompt them with 'an egg-cup full?' or' a tea-cup full?'. The reply will give some idea as to the severity of the bleed
• Was there any associated — change in the colour of your motions? (malaena) — loss of consciousness? — light-headedness?	Positive answers to these questions suggest that the bleed was a large one

Fact sheet: Essential questions in the assessment of haematemesis—cont'd

Essential questions	Clinical relevance
• Any previous swallowing problems?	Suggests an oesophageal cause. If the patient has progressive dysphagia this strongly suggests oesophageal carcinoma
• Any previous indigestion?	Suggests peptic ulceration
• Any recent weight loss?	Suggests cancer of the stomach or oesophagus. Some patients with gastric ulcers also lose a significant amount of weight
• Have you had previous problems with your stomach?	Peptic ulceration was a chronic relapsing disease before the advent of *H. pylori* eradication therapy. Patients who have had a previous partial gastrectomy are more prone to cancer in the gastric remnant. Patients with coeliac disease are more prone to gastric lymphoma and adenocarcinoma of the stomach and oesophagus
• What medicines are you taking? Have you taken any other medicines recently?	Patients taking NSAIDs and aspirin are at increased risk of developing peptic ulceration
• How much alcohol do you take?	An accurate alcohol history is mandatory. A Mallory–Weiss tear frequently follows an alcoholic binge. Patients who chronically abuse alcohol may develop cirrhosis and oesophageal varices

31

Haemoptysis

Mr. George Brearley is a 72-year-old man with a history of haemoptysis. Take a history to identify possible causes.

Essential skills required

- Knowledge of causes of haemoptysis and ability to differentiate between them.
- Ability to obtain relevant information.
- Focussed approach.
- Identify and deal with potentially serious causes of haemoptysis.

Think list

Your agenda	Mr. Brearley's agenda
• Obtain clear focussed history.	• Thinks it may be related to smoking.
• Identify serious causes of haemoptysis.	• Concerned that this may be something serious.
• Address any questions or anxieties.	

Danger! Common pitfalls

There are several common mistakes which students make that can be easily avoided.

✗ Not checking prior understanding.
✗ Lack of basic knowledge.
✗ Insensitive handling of a scary situation.
✗ Ignoring Mr. Brearley's agenda.

It is vital that you deal with the patient sensitively and considerately. Coughing up blood is a terrifying experience for any patient, especially as most people will worry it means they have cancer. Patients may try to down play the severity in the hope that it will settle. Likewise, they may be unkeen to admit they smoke, for fear of being judged.

Sometimes it is easier asking, 'How much do you smoke' rather than 'Do you smoke?'.

Patients asked, 'How much do you smoke?' would assume you are a clever doctor who could already tell they were a smoker. There's no point in hiding anything from you! If they do not smoke, follow up with 'Have you ever smoked?' just to check on exposure.

The fact sheet below outlines the causes of haemoptysis. Remember that chronic obstructive pulmonary disease is not a cause of haemoptysis. Younger non-smokers presenting with this symptom often have negative investigations, with no cause found. Despite this, the most important diagnosis to consider is lung cancer.

You may be required to discuss likely investigations for haemoptysis. In particular, you should be able to explain the procedure of bronchoscopy. This is covered in detail earlier in the book.

Fact sheet: Causes of haemoptysis

- Lung cancer
- Benign lung tumour
- Pneumonia—usually *Pneumococcus* spp
- Pulmonary tuberculosis
- Pulmonary embolus
- Bronchiectasis
- Acute left ventricular failure

Fact sheet: Essential questions in the assessment of haemoptysis

Essential questions	Clinical relevance
• Tell me what has been happening to you.	Nice open question to start with
• Are you sure you coughed up the blood and didn't vomit it up?	Some patients find it difficult to differentiate between haemoptysis and haematemesis
• What does your sputum look like?	Purulent green sputum with blood in it or rust-coloured sputum suggests a pneumonia or tuberculosis. Frank blood suggests a cancer or bronchiectasis. The bleeding in the latter condition is usually bright red and may be of large volume. Frothy white sputum tinged with pink suggests pulmonary oedema due to left ventricular failure

Fact sheet: Essential questions in the assessment of haemoptysis—cont'd

Essential questions	Clinical relevance
• Have you had any breathlessness?	It is important to distinguish acute from chronic onset of breathlessness. All the common causes of haemoptysis can cause breathlessness. Pulmonary embolus and left ventricular failure usually cause acute dyspnoea
• Have you had any chest pain, and what was it like?	Pleuritic pain suggests pulmonary embolus or pneumonia. Patients with lung cancer may have bony pain from rib metastases
• What illnesses have you had in the past?	A history of myocardial infarction or valvular heart disease/rheumatic fever suggests left ventricular failure. Patients with bronchiectasis may have a history of whooping cough as a child
• How much do you smoke?	Current and past smoking history is mandatory. Smokers have a life-time risk of up to 1 in 10 of developing lung cancer
• Alcohol history	Pulmonary tuberculosis is more common in alcoholics and immigrants

32

Abdominal pain

Mrs. Samantha Sprott is a 46-year-old woman who attended the emergency department with abdominal pain. Take a history to identify possible causes.

Essential skills required

- Knowledge of causes of abdominal pain and ability to differentiate between them.
- Ability to obtain relevant information.
- Focussed approach.
- Identify and deal with potentially serious causes of abdominal pain.

Think list

Your agenda
- Obtain clear focussed history.
- Identify serious causes of abdominal pain.
- Address any questions or anxieties.

Mrs. Sprott's agenda
- She thinks she has got appendicitis.
- Concerned that this may be something serious.

Danger! Common pitfalls

There are several common mistakes which students make that can be easily avoided.

✗ Not checking prior understanding.
✗ Lack of basic knowledge.
✗ Unsystematic approach.
✗ Ignoring Mrs. Sprott's agenda.

The fact sheet on page 206 outlines causes of abdominal pain. The first thing to do is establish the site of the pain, as the common causes of abdominal pain are different, depending on the location of the pain. Once you have established whether the pain is upper, mid or lower abdominal in position, you need to then tailor your questions to the differential diagnosis in the fact sheet below using the questions outlined in the following fact sheet.

Fact sheet: Causes of abdominal pain

Upper	Mid	Lower

• Peptic ulcer
• Pancreatitis
• Gallstone disease
• Stomach cancer
• Pancreatic cancer
• Liver metastases
• Non-ulcer dyspepsia
• Above diaphragm:
  — pulmonary embolus
  — chest infection
  — cardiac
	• Aortic aneurysm
	• Small bowel obstruction
	• Any cause of upper or lower abdominal pain
		• Appendicitis
		• Renal colic
		• Diverticulitis
		• Strangulated hernia
		• Crohn's disease
		• Constipation
		• Colonic obstruction
		• Ischaemic colitis
		• Urinary tract infection
		• Gynaecological:
		  — ovarian cyst
		  — ectopic pregnancy
		  — pelvic infection

Fact sheet: Essential questions in the assessment of abdominal pain

Essential questions	Clinical relevance
• Where do you feel the pain worst?	This will help frame your differential diagnosis as set out in fact sheet above
• Pain can be a difficult thing to describe. Using your own words how would you describe it?	Colicky pain is seen in obstruction to a hollow viscus, e.g.: • bile duct—upper abdomen • ureter—loin to groin • small bowel—mid abdomen • large bowel—lower abdomen
• Does the pain move anywhere?	Radiation to: • shoulder tip is seen in diaphragmatic irritation, e.g. cholecystitis. • groin is seen in renal colic • back is seen in aortic aneurysm and pancreatic disease
• Did the pain start suddenly?	Abrupt onset suggests stones, AAA, acute obstruction

Fact sheet: Essential questions in the assessment of abdominal pain—cont'd

Essential questions	Clinical relevance
• Have you had similar attacks of pain?	Paroxysmal upper abdominal pain in a middle-aged woman is gallstones until proven otherwise. Peptic ulcer disease waxes and wanes over weeks or months
• Does anything make the pain worse?	Pain aggravated by coughing suggests peritoneal irritation. Epigastric pain after meals suggests gastric ulceration
• Does anything make the pain better? • Do you have any other associated symptoms when you get the pain?	Rolling up in a ball often eases the pain of renal colic. Eating sometimes eases duodenal ulcer pain
• Are your bowels working properly?	Absolute constipation (including lack of flatus production) suggests bowel obstruction
• Have you lost any weight over recent weeks?	Significant weight loss is seen in malignant disease
• Any increased urinary frequency or pain on passing water?	Suggests urinary tract infection
• A full gynaecological history is mandatory in women with lower abdominal pain.	In particular, ask about last menstrual period, risk of pregnancy
• What illnesses/operations have you had in the past?	Patients with a partial gastrectomy are at increased risk of developing stomach cancer in the gastric remnant. Patients with coeliac disease are at increased risk of stomach and oesophageal adenocarcinoma as well as GI lymphoma
• What medicines are you taking? Have you taken any other medicines recently?	Patients taking NSAIDs are at risk of developing peptic ulceration
• Are there any illnesses that run in the family?	Crohn's disease has a genetic element

33

Rectal bleeding

Mr. Joachim Wilson is a 62-year-old man who complains of rectal bleeding. Take a history to identify possible causes.

Essential skills required

- Knowledge of causes of rectal bleeding and ability to differentiate between them.
- Ability to obtain relevant information.
- Focussed approach.
- Identify and deal with potentially serious causes of rectal bleeding.

Think list

Your agenda
- Obtain clear focussed history.
- Identify serious causes of rectal bleeding including chronic diseases.
- Address any questions or anxieties

Mr. Wilson's agenda
- Hopes he just has piles.
- Concerned that this may be something serious.
- Father died of colon cancer.

Danger! Common pitfalls

There are several common mistakes which students make that can be easily avoided.

- ✗ Not checking prior understanding.
- ✗ Lack of basic knowledge.
- ✗ Not anticipating potential need to break bad news.
- ✗ Ignoring Mr. Wilson's agenda.

The fact sheet on page 209 outlines the common causes of rectal bleeding. Remember that blood on the toilet paper when wiping is a very common symptom and is present in up to 20% of the population at any one time. If this is the only symptom it is highly unlikely that he has major underlying pathology.

Mr. Wilson is at an age where bowel cancer is more likely and an essential diagnosis to consider. Questions should focus on diagnosing or ruling out this as a cause of rectal bleeding. Whenever taking a history that may lead to a diagnosis of cancer, you must be prepared to discuss this possibility if asked to. In addition you may be required to explain likely tests the patient may require (such as colonoscopy). These aspects of the consultation are covered earlier in the book.

It is essential in clinical practice to perform a rectal examination on a patient who presents with rectal bleeding. The authors have seen numerous patients with advanced rectal cancer where this examination had been initially omitted and the symptoms ascribed to 'piles'.

Fact sheet: Causes of rectal bleeding

Anorectal	*Colonic*
• Piles	• Colonic Cancer
• Anal fissure	• Colonic polyp
• Rectal cancer	• Diverticular disease
• Rectal polyp	• Inflammatory bowel disease
• Proctitis	• Ischaemic colitis
• Solitary rectal ulcer	• Pseudomembranous colitis
• Idiopathic	

Fact sheet: Essential questions in the assessment of rectal bleeding

Essential questions	*Clinical relevance*
• I understand you have passed some blood from your back passage. Tell me in your own words what has been happening to you.	Nice open question to start with
• Is the blood just on the toilet paper?	This is a very common symptom and is found in people with piles, anal fissure and after vigorous wiping. If this is the patient's only symptom it is highly unlikely that he has any serious underlying pathology
• Is the blood mixed in with the stool, or just coating the outside?	The former is found in most causes with left-sided colonic pathology, the latter implies an anal or low rectal cause

Fact sheet: Essential questions in the assessment of rectal bleeding—cont'd	
Essential questions	*Clinical relevance*
• Any pain on opening the bowels?	Commonly found in an anal fissure
• Do you experience urgency, where you have to rush to the loo to open your bowels?	This usually implies significant pathology in the rectum or colon and is found in inflammatory bowel disease, and rectal cancer. In both these the rectum is poorly compliant, and when stool reaches this level it has to be expelled
• How often are you opening your bowels per day?	Patients with diarrhoea and rectal bleeding often have significant pathology, e.g. rectal cancer, inflammatory bowel disease. Current bowel habit needs to be compared to previous bowel habit. Remember that some people have their bowels open three times per day and this is normal for them
• Do you have to get out of bed to open your bowels?	This is very suggestive of significant colorectal pathology
• Any weight loss?	Suggestive of advanced malignancy, but also seen in inflammatory bowel disease
• Any mouth ulcers, new joint pains grittiness in the eyes?	These systemic symptoms are sometimes seen in inflammatory bowel disease
• Are there any bowel illnesses that run in the family?	Colorectal cancer and inflammatory bowel disease both have a genetic element

Note

Ischaemic colitis is usually found in the elderly. The patient has usually had another illness with a period of hypotension. They develop a relative ischaemia in the watershed area of the middle and inferior mesenteric arteries at the splenic flexure. This results in abdominal pain and a plum-coloured stool. It is usually self-limiting provided the patient is given appropriate supportive care and careful fluid balance.

    Pseudomembranous colitis is caused by infection with *C. difficile* spp. It usually follows treatment with broad-spectrum antibiotics such as clindamycin or a cephalosporin. The diarrhoea is sometimes bloody and extremely offensive to smell.

34

The nightmare scenario

Miss Jill Hubbert is an 18-year-old with a long history of asthma. She has been an inpatient many times in the past and is re-admitted with a severe exacerbation. On initial assessment she is clearly unwell and finds it difficult to complete sentences with one breath.

You have arranged a salbutamol nebuliser via high flow oxygen. What three questions should you ask that will influence your management?

This is a stinker of a question! We have only included it since, believe it or not, it has come up in the past and stumped candidates. Strictly speaking it doesn't test communication skills, although some examiners would argue differently. It's particularly unfair because it is testing whether you can guess what the examiner is thinking! However, the argument for the question being included is as follows.

Candidates need to be able to identify an unwell patient and in that situation, ask the bare essential questions that will direct appropriate care and intervention. Taking a long, detailed history from someone who is likely to expire without treatment is pointless. This asthmatic needs urgent treatment and any questions need to be focussed and appropriate. Don't forget, Miss Hubbert is extremely breathless and answering questions will be an effort.

Essential question number one

> **Doctor:** 'Have you ever been admitted to intensive care or needed to go on a machine to help your breathing?'

If this patient has ever been admitted to intensive care and/or needed ventilation you already know that she has the potential to 'go off big time'. Intensive care teams sometimes talk about the 'fester factor', which is the time doctors 'sit on' a sick patient before referring them to ITU. If there is a sick asthmatic in the hospital, they would like to know about them sooner rather than later. A patient with a previous ITU history should make you have a very low threshold for referral.

Essential question number two

> **Doctor:** 'What medicines have you taken for your asthma before coming into hospital?'

If this patient has a long history of asthma, she will have spent her childhood in and out of hospital and will be sick of the place. Young asthmatics will do anything to avoid coming into the hospital, especially as they know they are going to be subjected to arterial blood gases, which hurt. To avoid admission, they will have taken maximal therapy in the community. Many asthmatics won't come in until they have been on steroids for several days and taken hourly salbutamol nebulisers. You need to know what they have taken since it will give you an idea of what needs giving next.

Lets look at it another way: asthma guidelines will suggest we start with oxygen/nebuliser and then re-assess. However, a patient failing on salbutamol nebulisers and steroids in the community isn't going to improve on the same treatment in hospital. They need something added, such as aminophylline. Knowledge of previous recent medication will guide how quickly you should escalate the treatment.

Essential question number three

> **Doctor:** 'Are you taking a medicine called aminophylline?'

The next step in the treatment of this patient would be the introduction of a theophylline infusion. It is worth revising the pharmacology of aminophylline since it is an important emergency drug. You may recall that it has a narrow therapeutic window, which means that there isn't much difference between the treatment dose and the toxic dose. For aminophylline to work, a loading dose needs to be infused into the blood stream, followed by a maintenance dose. Patients already taking an oral theophylline do not need a loading dose since they already have a fair amount of the drug in their system. Giving a loading dose to someone already on aminophylline would make him or her toxic and liable to a fatal arrhythmia.

Likewise, if they are already taking aminophylline, you should have an even lower threshold for referral to ITU since you will have exhausted most therapeutic options on the open ward.

Index